A terrific book here full of insight, information a.... ..gµy interesting people...gives the book a warm and beating heart. This is a very important book...an insight into the fantastic variety of human responses to adversity.
-- **Gabrielle Lord, best-selling author**

Society is stretching the definition of mental health. As Tanveer notes, mental health has been equated with emotional distress. We are changing our view of trauma, seeking counsellors for all occasions. What's going on? Tanveer's case studies illuminate these trends. But readers will find them interesting for their own sake, stories of humanity. His book is nothing less than an account of how we live now: from Mujahideen to Mcmansions.
-- **Bob Carr, former NSW Premier**

Tanveer Ahmed's Fragile Nation comes as revelation to me. I have following his writing for many years and have always been impressed by his knowledge, valuable insights and willingness to express unpopular truths. But I was riveted by his stories of the people he cares for as a psychiatrist working in Western Sydney: angry white men, alienated youth seduced by Islam, damaged refugees, the children of tiger mothers. Amazing people revealed with sensitivity and candour, blessedly free of the ideological claptrap that often captures the saintly souls who work in the helping professions. Here's to Tanveer Ahmed – Australia's Theodore Dalrymple.
-- **Bettina Arndt, author and clinical psychologist.**

Dr Ahmed argues clearly and forcefully for a less mechanistic and bureaucratic psychiatry, which harms our culture and society as well as individuals. His book will be unwelcome in the very circles where it is most needed.
--**Theodore Dalrymple, UK Psychiatrist and Author**

This is a fantastic read. Fragile Nation offers a compelling account of the way that culture, morality and psychology intersect and influence individual behaviour in a transnational world.
-- **Frank Furedi, author and emeritus professor of sociology at the University of Kent, United Kingdom**

Tanveer Ahmed is a Sydney based psychiatrist working in private practice. He lives with his wife and two daughters. His first book is a migration memoir titled *The Exotic Rissole*.

# FRAGILE NATION

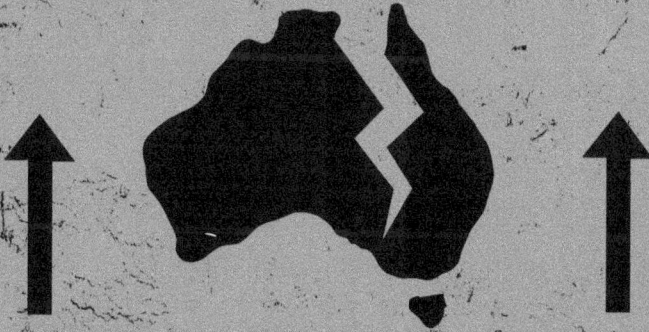

## VULNERABILITY, RESILIENCE AND VICTIMHOOD

## TANVEER AHMED

Connor Court Publishing

Published in 2016 by Connor Court Publishing Pty Ltd

Connor Court Publishing Pty Ltd
PO Box 7257
Redland Bay QLD 4165
sales@connorcourt.com

www.connorcourt.com

Phone  0497-900-685

Printed in Australia

ISBN: 978-1-925501-34-6


Front cover design:  Josh Durham

*The patient stories are based on my personal experience and memories of cases. Names and details have been changed.*

"We imagine that human nature doesn't change. We like to say that but I don't think it's true because we have, in the course of the centuries, altered ourselves."

Theodore Zeldin, Oxford Professor of History

# CONTENTS

Introduction 9

Marginal Man 15

Closet Gays 33

Fragile Nation 51

On Purity 69

Secular Priests 87

Angry White Men 109

Mujahideen to Mcmansions 127

The Trouble With Teenagers 143

Brick Lane in Lakemba 165

Why Addiction is like a Love Affair 187

Conclusion 203

Acknowledgements 207

References 209

# INTRODUCTION

I knew being a psychiatrist was for me when, as a medical student on my first day in a mental health facility, I found myself tackling a patient with two burly security guards. The patient was trying to escape a locked hospital ward because he thought the staff were aliens trying to poison him. This was not altogether delusional, given the nurses' outfits were purple pyjamas and he was being injected with unpronounceable medications. But that a person's mind could play such tricks intrigued me, more so than the workings of bodily organs.

Years later I treat patients in multiple arenas, from my main practice in western Sydney with its mix of immigrants, tradesmen and service workers to visiting jails to determine if clients are mad or bad to flying on wobbly planes to regional Australia. I remain as fascinated with the human experience as the first day I was chasing a fugitive patient.

This book incorporates patient cases with personal history and social analysis. It is an extension of that wonder in a job that British psychologist Adam Phillips writes "reveals with scientific sobriety the slapstick of ordinary life."

The patients reveal the extraordinary range of responses to emotional distress, from the atheist who starts praying excessively to the computer programmer throwing his clothes off in the middle of a car park. The cultural rise in mental health comes at a time when life's project has shifted to self-fulfillment via individual psychology. This puts enormous pressure on us all to forever fine tune our psychological well-being.

There have been dramatic improvements in the treatment and stigma surrounding mental illness but it has also reached a stage where the term mental health is a synonym for emotional distress. I worry that excessive promotion of human fragility in the face of adversity risks enfeebling those we seek to help. It also risks corrupting public debate by framing minority groups as too vulnerable to be engaged as citizens.

The chapters comprise essays and patient cases relating to specific themes. They vary from the enormous growth of post-traumatic stress disorder and how this is changing our relationship with adversity to how a quest for purity and authenticity are influencing both religious fundamentalism and our greater consumption of alternative medicine.

The patients profiled tend to be from different cultural groups. This transcultural cross section represents my interests and the demography of my practice in outer Sydney.

Groups from traditional cultures are asked to alter their view of themselves drastically when confronted with mental illness from seeing themselves as relational beings tied to clan, family and tradition to a view which sees them primarily as individuals with a private, personal realm.

The psychological sciences promise a way of helping people realize their individuality through examining their desires and instincts, much of which had previously been consciously inaccessible. They have helped illuminate the ethical battles of daily living, arising first in relation to parents and ending with our confrontation with death.

The history of psychology helped lay the foundations for many of the upheavals of the twentieth century, from the consumer society to recognition of minority groups- women, blacks and homosexuals.

Just as we live in disruptive times, this also affects our conceptions of human nature, which are in flux. I argue in this book that we have an opportunity to incorporate a sophisticated view of human nature that merges the wisdom of our ancestors promulgated through religious and moral systems with the great advances we have made in our understanding of the psychological sciences.

Chapter One called Marginal Man looks at young Muslims grappling with their identity and then expressing it through new versions of Islam. The trend has overlaps with religious revivalism among other ethnic groups trying to be both modern but not overtly Western.

The second chapter looks at the conflicted lives of closet gay men and my experience in attending their support group. The cases are a reminder of the challenges many people still have in escaping the context of their families and traditional communities. It's also a hint that closet gays have a greater influence in our culture than we might imagine, from Catholic priests to debates around transgender issues.

Chapter three titled "Fragile Nation" examines cases of post-traumatic stress disorder and the loosening of its definition. Through the stories of the patients our changing attitudes to adversity and suffering is illustrated. I contend that there is a growing risk of painting people as fragile which is disempowering them from achieving recovery.

The fourth story incorporating a patient who retreats into a warped idea of healthy food and its overlaps with our search for purity looks at our greater emphasis on subjective feelings. The relationship to our views on authenticity is examined and how this can isolate us psychologically. The rise in virtuous food and alternative medicine is a search for the transcendent at a time when liberalism can feel without an uplifting vision.

The fifth chapter is a look at how so many moral questions previously falling under the realm of religion now come to the sector of mental health. It also asks at what stage does treating illness become performance enhancement, as the explosion of mental illness diagnosis might imply.

Chapter 6 titled "Angry White Men" looks at some of the psychological undercurrents among the white working class from fatherlessness to the nostalgia for the local. It ties in patient cases who were involved with anti-immigration groups. I argue that learned helplessness is a common state among such groups but the resentment is channeled externally.

Stories of refugee patients incorporate one chapter and outline their extraordinary journeys from war and exile. Their trends in consuming mental health are fascinating for they are usually from cultures with little emphasis on individual psychology. The trauma they have often experienced is beyond our imagination yet some struggle more in the day to day battles of Australian resettlement.

A chapter on adolescent mental health asks the question whether teenagers have unique, heightened pressures today given there is much evidence that mental disorder has risen among them, particularly self harm. I argue that the greater focus on positive feelings has helped make the next generation less able to tolerate uncomfortable, negative emotions that are part and parcel of daily life.

Chapter 9 is a look through one specific case at the women who arrive in Australia through arranged marriage and the isolation they can face. The clash in expectations is highlighted but more universal changes in romantic relationships is also illustrated.

The final chapter looks at addiction in different cultural groups and asks whether we have ever lived in a time with a greater access to novelty and substances. I contend that addiction is a good example of a combination of moral and psychological factors, a special kind of voluntary activity. I also argue that modern inequality is driven greatly by variations in psychological skills.

While the book is ultimately a series of topics illustrated through patient cases, there are political themes. I contend that factors such as the greater construction of human vulnerability and the rise of feelings as an arbiter of objective truth have combined to promote the rise of subjectivity in our discourse. This threatens the idea of autonomous, reasoned individuals at the centre of our polity and self-knowledge as the universal aspiration of Man.

But my patients and their extraordinary courage and grace in the face of tremendous adversity remain at the core of the narrative. I hope their wide variety of responses to crafting a meaningful life at a time when the old certainties and structures have crumbled will inform and inspire.

# 1

# Marginal Man

The psychology of beards is not something I received training in either as a medical student or as a psychiatric trainee. There were no world experts giving us lectures on the symbolism of the beard as a marker of identity or an assertion of masculinity. The search for authenticity in the form of manicured, managed dishevelment was not predicted by social researchers. But here it was in my rooms.

The carefully groomed beard rarely presented in outer metropolitan areas, given its distance from the cultural centres of the inner city, the boroughs mimicking the hipster Meccas such as Williamsburg in New York. There were no cafes in Blacktown with signs like "Come in hungry, leave feeling edgy." Facial hair in my patients arose out of neglect or successful charity drives like Movember.

But it had interesting connotations and meanings in patients from traditional cultural groups, particularly Muslims but sometimes others such as Sikhs.

Jamil was a patient I had treated for many years, since he was aged fifteen. Raised in a Pakistani family, his parents were well educated and culturally religious, in that they weren't particularly devout but attended mosque on special events such as the end of Ramadan. I took considerable satisfaction in seeing Jamil for what were now annual check-ups. He was due to complete university in accounting and had already found a job for a major firm. His parents were gushing at every appointment, bringing in gifts and food. I was particularly fond of a semolina- based sweet known as halwa, which the Pakistanis did better than anybody else. Jamil's mother would send an annual supply packaged neatly in a lunch box, carried in by Jamil.

But it was not always so. He first presented in his late teens barely able to attend school. Suffering panic attacks at the beginning of Year 11, struggling with bad acne and feeling socially inept as playground complexities were magnified, Jamil declined psychologically and started having thoughts of self-harm. Referred by the school counsellor, his initial presentation seemed much like other adolescents suffering social anxiety.

We used to think adolescence was no different to adulthood psychologically, but this view has been firmly disproven by scientific studies. The psychiatrist Erik Erikson is renowned for suggesting each stage of life carried with it a task of maturation, an obstacle necessary to progress to the next stage, almost like a real life, psychological video game. In the middle years of adulthood the conflict is called intimacy versus isolation in reference to our search for some kind of close partner.

During our latter decades, once the demands of child rearing and career were overcome, the stage was called generativity versus stagnation. Those who were unable to find ways to give their skills and experience to younger generations struggled to come to terms with the final chapters of their lives.

In adolescence the key task, according to Erikson, was known as identity versus role diffusion. Your mission, if you chose to accept it, was to start forming a sense of who you were beyond your parents, which was inevitably your key relationship up until that time. It was a time to build autonomy. As teenagers we did this through our relationships in our peer group, which is why there was no more powerful time in terms of how self-conscious we were.

It is no coincidence that so many movies have been made about the high school experience. There is also evidence that we carry our self-image formed in the playground, to a large extent, for the rest of our lives. So the athletic jock popular with girls who ends up failing high school and working in a not so salubrious job still walks around like he is the alpha male. Likewise the nerdy intellectual with obscure interests who may have been teased and shunned by prospective members of the opposite sex, still carried around the chip on the shoulder even after becoming, say, the CEO of a multinational or the Prime Minister.

Social anxiety is most pronounced during this adolescent period and was characterized by the fear that you are not good enough and might be exposed, socially humiliated, in the event you were scrutinised. The fear was experienced as virtually mortal by sufferers in what they worried was a kind of social death. Scrutiny could come in seemingly harmless forms – being casually looked at, being asked for an opinion or, more threateningly, to perform in some way, such as in a sporting endeavour or academic task.

The fear manifested in panic attacks, anticipation of further panic attacks and if things worsened, an increasing range of avoidance behaviours culminating in no longer being able to attend school. What is known in the field as school refusal is regarded as an emergency, for it threatens healthy social and intellectual development.

This is exactly how Jamil presented. Much of his history was no different from other adolescents. Except for one aspect. He started growing a beard. It began as an experiment. He worried it might get dirty and smell of his mother's curry. The beard also shielded some of his acne.

He bought an electrical trimmer to keep it better groomed and started shampooing it in the weeks before first consulting with me, although it was still overhanging his chest.

The change in his appearance coincided with him becoming more religious, something he shared with some of his Pakistani family friends. They read Koranic passages together at Sunday school, sent stories of the Prophet Muhammad to each other on social media and during school holidays met at the mosque for Friday prayer. The behaviour did not worry Jamil's parents initially, although they did not share his convictions. They bragged to their friends that he could read the Koran with perfect Arabic pronunciation, engaging his throat skilfully for the more guttural sounds and touching his tongue on the roof of his mouth for a 'dh' sound. They saw it as positive, something that might protect him from the potential temptations of sex and drugs at school and the Western social context.

Patients like Jamil were very close to home. I was raised in a not too dissimilar household, one from South Asia with loving parents eager for me to have a good education while also maintaining strong links with my ancestral culture. This resistance to change manifested in a determined opposition to any kind of integration with Western culture. While I too rebelled against this attachment to the past, with maturity I recognised that my parents had a reasonable fear that without their resistance our cultural traditions would simply be wiped out in a generation.

Different households had different devotion to religious practices, reflecting some of the tensions from the home countries.

For example, whereas Pakistan was founded as an Islamic state after partition from India in 1947, Bangladesh split from Pakistan in 1971 to preserve its linguistic identity.

While Pakistan had a sizeable and sophisticated intelligentsia who were more likely to migrate overseas, they were also among the most conservative with regards to their views around Islamic practice, reflected in multiple international surveys which showed Pakistani nationals held considerable sympathies with Islamic State, the Charlie Hebdo killers and the aims of terrorism.

The Deobandi brand of Islam borne from the resentments resulting from British colonialism bred a hostile, oppositional religious practice that had strong synergies with Islamism. A century later large numbers of British citizens involved in terrorism-related activities have had links to Deobandi organisations or mosques.

Being a Muslim dissident is something of a family business. My maternal grandfather was the only openly atheist in his entire region on the Bangladeshi-Indian border, a considerable rarity over half a century ago. As a child he witnessed the slaughter in the name of religious fervour that partition wrought, in which over a million people were killed. Throughout his life he spoke out about what he felt was the misguided nature of religious belief, despite having a younger brother who was a mullah. He viewed religious practice as a type of status seeking, particularly convenient for those who had failed in worldly endeavours but who could then adopt a high tone and berate others for their focus on material or professional success. This was often the attraction to becoming a village mullah.

The key tension during Bangladeshi independence was around the forces of secular humanism and religious fundamentalism. While the forces of humanism may have won out, religious tensions have never been far from the surface, most recently illustrated by the tragic terrorist acts in the capital city, Dhaka, where twenty people were killed in an upmarket bakery. Those same tensions spill out into the suburbs of Sydney, such as through archaic organisations celebrating past leaders or in dinner party bust-ups.

But the overall trend in current generations of Muslims is towards greater religiosity, which is not necessarily the same as religion. It tends to refer to the self-expression or an individual formulation of religious faith and practice, with overlaps to people who deny being religious but say they are spiritual. Religiosity has a greater focus on the self. Religion could be considered as a more coherent set of beliefs managed by professional holders of that knowledge, namely priests and theologians.

Well before the age of terror was announced spectacularly via the World Trade Centre attacks, I observed friends around me becoming unusually religious, wearing beards and hijabs, despite being from families who were not particularly pious. I found it a curious trend and wanted to participate but struggled to believe in the Koran as the word of God. The ideas were so contradictory and obviously aimed at nomadic tribes in sixth century Arabia. The idea of applying the set of ideas as the foundation for living amid the complexities of modern life seemed absurd. I would shake my head when I heard arguments among family friends about whether we should use toothpaste that contained traces of pig fat or avoid mixing with non-Muslims for fear of being morally corrupted. Our community wanted to have their cake and eat it too, in that they were more than happy to enjoy the benefits of greater material prosperity but were resistant to the prospect of having to engage and perhaps acquire any social and cultural characteristics of their adopted land.

Households tended to preach the virtues of tradition, segregation of the sexes and communalism, whereas the outside world preached the opposite. I could understand how this might seem like a cultural assault to my parents and relatives. The challenge was how to reach a compromise between the old and the new but instead the reaction by some was a defensive retreat into even greater traditionalism or religiosity.

It was not a surprise that many children growing up in such a contradictory environment found the formation of a coherent identity, the key task of adolescence, challenging. This formation is hard enough without the cultural complexities given the rapid changes in family structure, the rise of meritocracy and technology.

During a trip to Britain as a medical student, I met psychologists who worked with South Asians growing up in the United Kingdom, namely those from Indian, Bangladeshi and Pakistani families. They had higher rates of mental illness compared to the broader British population, particularly in young women. The rate was likely to have been even higher given the greater stigma around mental health in such groups.

The sociologist Everett Stonequist coined the term "marginal man" in referring to people who were caught between two distinct cultural systems. He used the term in reference to the mass migration occurring between the world wars, but they apply even more so to today. The marginal man straddles multiple cultures in the same society but may feel rejected or disconnected from both or all of them. The threats to identity may then manifest in greater levels of deviance. This is particularly true for many children who can barely speak their parents' language and have limited access to their ancestral cultures.

The emotional distress may present through bouts of

depression, self-harm or anxiety disorders. Boys were more likely to externalise their distress and act out, reflected by their greater numbers in the British criminal justice system. The rates would almost certainly be lower in Australia given the strict selection and skilled migration background of the same ethnic groups. South Asians in Australia commonly have medical, computer or accounting backgrounds or if they arrived more recently completed a degree or diploma locally before becoming citizens. Those in Britain migrated on mass to work in textile factories after World War II. The refugee derived groups in Australia such as the Lebanese or Afghans are more comparable to British South Asians in terms of their class and educational backgrounds.

In attempting to cope with their psychological strain one way such youth can maintain a coherent identity is to attach their self-image to a group with strong, structured beliefs and rules.

The trends in Britain coincided with the greater religiosity I was seeing among my peers in the community. A pointer to such trends piqued my interest in the specialty of psychiatry. It was a unique aspect of modernity that such disparate groups from such traditional, clan-based backgrounds were suddenly thrust into very different societies and asked to get on with it, especially at a time when there was such rapid social change fostered by the explosion in communications technologies.

Jamil was an exception in that he presented to mental health services. He had his own vulnerabilities, which tipped him over the edge. His earliest memory was of his parents panicking around his older brother who suffered from life-threatening asthma. Shy, softly spoken and socially awkward, Jamil had a greater tendency to internalise distress. But the vast majority of young Muslims who veer towards religious observance do so as a reasonable adaptation to their circumstances, a more culturally acceptable version of adolescent rebellion. If they were white they might have become punks or goths and pierced their nose and nipples, but instead they don hijabs and prayer hats and grow beards.

The Pew Survey has repeatedly shown that virtually every ethnic or religious group become less religious after migrating to the West, except for Muslims who as a group tend to become more religious. In spite of some aspects of Muslim behaviour being cultural expressions of broader patterns, there also appear to be some unique trends peculiar to the Islamic community.

French academic Olivier Roy in his book *Globalised Islam* writes of the notion of identity Islam, a modern version of Islamic practice undertaken by Muslims growing up in the West. They are unique in history in that their practice of Islam is de-territorialised – not tied to any geography or pre-existing culture. This is where they are in fact rebelling against their parents' version of religious practice which they perceive as stained by cultural traditions. Their parents' combination of culture, nationalism and religion were not in opposition, unlike those growing up in countries like Australia or Britain.

The rejection of culture is central to the notion, for they believe there is a true Islam that exists pristine and pure stripped from any cultural strains. This is arguably a fiction for no religion can exist without a local, cultural dimension, but not unlike others trying to find stronger links with nature through food or medicine, it was another version of a search for purity.

I would often have long chats with Jamil as he began to improve and was interested in his religious views. He spoke of his attachment to the "ummah", which referred to the international community of believers. It was an imagined community but he felt it strongly, identifying with the Palestinians and even Bosnians in Eastern Europe. What did he have in common with

Slavs in the Eastern Bloc I wondered? But in a time of a diluted notion of community, it was this kind of imagined community that held appeal. I also couldn't help thinking that the notion of a global, oppressed class of Muslims from Palestine to France to the Philippines sounded awfully like the international working class motif of Marxism. During my conversations with Jamil sometimes I felt like Lenin had been reincarnated as a skinny Pakistani boy who also liked Kanye West.

American sociologist Marcia Hermansen ran a study almost a decade ago looking at Muslim youth across American university campuses. What she found was that Muslim religiosity was primarily a defence mechanism to ward off the hurt of unbelonging. She writes:

> One can imagine the problems of Muslim youth, often isolated by having distinctive names, physical appearance, and being associated with a stigmatized culture and religion. No wonder the concept that they were actually the superior ones, fending off the corrupt and evil society around them, rang pleasant.

It was a bit like breaking up first with a boyfriend or girlfriend fearing they were about to break up with you. Instead of feeling rejected by mainstream society, Muslims through their religiosity rejected the mainstream. Theirs was a social protest. Rather than feeling socially awkward, unattractive or unable to mix, they could believe they were morally superior and project any sense of hurt outwards through accusations of racism and discrimination. This is not to say such mistreatment doesn't exist, but there is plenty of evidence to suggest the rejection and self-segregation begins with Muslims first.

The positive is that such oppositionality and sense of protest, much like other kinds of adolescent rebellion tends to weaken as they become adults and acquire social mobility. This is particularly the case in countries like Australia, where skilled migrants have considerable social mobility and rise rapidly through the ranks of education and income. The weakening may be less pronounced in refugee-derived groups, which represent almost the entire supply of the hundred or so recruits Australia has had in terrorism-related activities, but the majority of them also rise, particularly in latter generations.

For Jamil this was expressed through a steady shortening of his beard. He was able to return to school rapidly with medications and counselling. While he struggled socially, he was able to score a good mark and gain entry into a prestigious accounting course. Despite having some involvement with the university Islamic society, he channelled his religious behaviour through visits to the mosque and occasional prayer meetings with other Muslims, mainly his family friends of Pakistani origin. He was also planning a Hajj trip to Mecca with some of his friends, a practice that was historically enacted by those in the final stages of their lives but is now common among Muslim youth living in the West. Mecca tour operators were going gangbusters. It sounded to me much like a Muslim version of a boy's trip away, but it was that little bit harder to question for his family and partners because it was bound up with God and religion. The bonding occurred through prayer and not alcohol.

Jamil continued to harbour strong anti-Western attitudes, primarily political. His faith was utterly stained with the grievance politics of the day. Once again having much in common with other left wing ideologies, he believed American imperialism was the root of all evil and held up writers like Middle East correspondent Robert Fisk and John Pilger as his intellectual heroes.

It was not my job to challenge his political views unless I

thought they overlapped with any kind of mental illness. His beard continued to shorten to the point where he noted it was effectively a goatee and could be interpreted as a fashion statement, although other Muslims would interpret it as an appropriate act of faith. Whereas the longer beard was a visible act of social protest and a firm identification of tribal belonging, the shorter goatee gave a much more subtle signal both to mainstream society and Muslims. It was a symbolic act of integration.

But I still found it frustrating that Jamil exhibited a trait I observed in other Muslims I met outside my practice, a refusal to accept there is anything particularly great or exceptional about Western society. He was raised to believe it was morally corrupt and saw the incredible achievements of human freedom in terms of licentiousness and a path to excessive inequality. Any of the positives such as women's rights or scientific achievements, he was quick to make questionable arguments that Islam did it first. The only way he might accept the positives of Western society was that if he could somehow convince himself that it was also, or even originally, "Islamic".

The one area he was beginning to celebrate as having been derived from the West was double entry bookkeeping, a result of his prowess and success as an accountant. I was pleased that his attachment was shifting from Allah and the ummah to the God of the audit.

I used to think trends I saw in patients like Jamil were unique to the Muslim community, but my views have changed. There is a kind of religious revivalism attractive to many young people. You only need to look at the extraordinary growth of the evangelical, Hillsong Church for example. Other churches would kill to have that kind of popularity and particularly the much younger cohort of followers.

I have had several patients over the years who presented with a variety of mental health problems, often related to childhood trauma or neglect, but after they joined Hillsong or another evangelical movement, I did not hear from them again. They basically recovered after finding purpose and belonging in a charismatic movement with a strong set of rules and structures. The patients usually had traits of black and white thinking. People were either good or bad and actions were right or wrong. This was common in what is known in mental health as personality disorder. But strict interpretations and tribal belonging combined with the expression of the individual self are things evangelical Christianity and identity Islam have in common.

A casual visit to a local church will illustrate the changing demographics. The modern Christian will increasingly have an Asian or black face and may be attracted to evangelical or Pentecostal forms of observances. Several of the local churches in the inner west of Sydney have been handed over to Korean or Chinese congregations. Drive further to outer metropolitan areas and they are just as likely to be packed to the brim with Pacific Islanders beautifully dressed in their Sunday best.

I have had several friends of Chinese origin who trained as doctors but became missionaries to live in places like Africa or regional China. While it's not quite going to Syria to fight for the Caliphate, these acts could also be considered as a kind of protest against modern, consumer life.

Indian author Pankaj Mishra writes in his book Temptations of the West of the various ways people in the subcontinent come to terms with modernity, particularly in negotiating the assault by American culture and materialism. Much of this is voraciously consumed, by the rapidly enriched middle classes, but there is still an attempt to exert a modern identity without it being perceived as merely a mimicking of bourgeois Westerners. Mishra's characters vary from aspiring Bollywood film actresses to Hindu nationalists, but they are all variations on this theme.

A similar process of projecting an outward image more easily perceived as modern occurs among ethnic groups living in the West, where they are on the search for self-expression that is not mimicry of the mainstream but nor do they want to revert to the habits and worldview of their parents, which is seen as nostalgic and of the past. Whether they don on a baseball cap and sprout lyrics from the latest rap star or grow a beard and mouth platitudes from a YouTube mullah, the process has considerable overlaps.

Religious observance through outer markers such as beards, pilgrimages to Mecca or transcendent ceremonies like a mass prayer or passionate, Gospel singing are a way of asserting such modern identities. There can be a born again quality about it, often beginning in young adulthood but maintained in a diluted version in later years as burgeoning families and career converge.

One aspect of working in mental health is its interface with the law, a necessity given so many people in our jails have mental health problems. I regularly visit correctional centres across the state to give opinions about how mad or bad some inmates are. Images of the religiously devout are hardly the stereotypes conjured up for most people when they think of prisoners, but it can be an interesting environment to observe born again Christians and Muslims.

Jails are a throwback, a kind of institutionalization that reminds me of psychiatric asylums. There can be a tension between punishment and rehabilitation in the setting of incarceration, but it's difficult not see an aim as the slow deadening of the spirit, designed to numb inmates and reduce the risk of accelerated tension and violence. The staff are often as institutionalised as the inmates.

In today's jails there is an emphasis on greater freedom for inmates, access to nature and possibility of training which has helped manage inmates, but the experience for visitors like me is often one of great irritation. Retinal scans, long checks of identity, the clang and slam of door after door, only to wait in yet another room with the same checks and questions.

Unlike my private rooms where I was more likely to see ethnic groups from professional backgrounds, jails are populated by the white, indigenous and ethnic underclass. The social organisation also descends into tribal, ethnic lines – the Lebs, the Abos, the Islanders.

The Muslims I see in jail have usually been antisocial for years, often involved in gangs or outlaw, motorcycle clubs and had little interest in religion before incarceration. I see them in old, craggy rooms usually at a small wooden table on the verge of breaking apart. The inmates arrive in green uniforms to be subjected to my interview. Unlike Jamil, they were usually from very different backgrounds, such as Lebanese or Iraqi. Compared to the softer, bookish traits I knew of South Asians, they had a more hyper-masculine, macho air, a greater tendency for bravado and displays of anger.

One man I visited was referred for a de-radicalisation program after he assaulted someone and called him a "Shiite prick". He was Lebanese but of the Sunni sect. His anger was aroused after his victim didn't have enough money to pay for a burger. Before long, after a series of text and social media messages, a brawl erupted at a local train station. The client had a history of drug use which is why I was asked to give an opinion, but it was curious that the reference to Shiites triggered a referral to a de-radicalisation program that was basically little more than a Sheik visiting the jail to go over some passages in the Koran and an occasional visit to an external counsellor to help him better manage anger. This was not unreasonable but was better described as a treatment protocol rather than the fancy title of deradicalisation.

While I have only had a handful of cases that overlapped with religious extremism, several clients became outwardly religious after starting a jail sentence, having spent much of their pre-jail years in the street, rebel identity mediated through hip hop culture. This unusual confluence has been referred to as 'jihadi-street', merging youth rebellion with Islamism. Like Jamil, outward markers such as long beards or eating Halal meat was both an expression of identity and an acceptable form of social protest, given it was perceived as the antithesis of the mainstream. Some clients admitted they only converted to Islam in jail to get better food. Their conversion was also an external signal of transformation, a prerequisite for redemption.

Despite being of Muslim parentage the social class of most of the inmates meant the dynamics of their families were very different from the skilled migrant of my family and ethnic community. Families were inevitably large and the parents had limited education, having migrated from rural villages decades before during Lebanon's civil war. The parenting style placed few limits on the boys yet strictly controlled the girls. The girls from such families were often more successful with regards to employment and education and rebelled against the constraints of their culture, caught between the misogyny of their ancestry and hyper-masculine but worldly failure of their male peers. The much propagated notion of the subjugated, submissive female is a rarity among second and third generation Muslims regardless of class or ethnicity. This can have its drawbacks, sometimes dangerously so in the form of domestic violence when males lash out against the threat of losing their power or fears that female assertion might be perceived as equivalent to sexual promiscuity within the community.

My patients from Muslim backgrounds whether or not they were in jail were particularly challenging. The marginal man scenario existed across all cultures, but those from non-Muslim background were not so vulnerable to latching on to the black and white, destructive thinking of Islamism. Muslims were among the most prone to projecting their problems outwards. If there was one region of the world where fields such as psychology and psychoanalysis have had the least penetration, it would be the Middle East.

There was considerable variation in how people viewed themselves and how strong their ties were to any kind of Muslim or ethnic community, especially after some had absorbed Western norms. But there was some truth in the much-criticised book *The Arab Mind* by anthropologist Raphael Patai who argues that shame and honour make up the moral axis of Arabs. Guilt, sin and redemption are closer to the axis of the Christian spectrum and allow an easier shift to the notion of an internal, psychological experience.

Modern ideologies such as communism and Islamism have their roots in the denial of the individual and, in turn, the significance of any private, psychological realm. Modern identity politics with its focus on sections of the community who are constructed as broadly vulnerable and encouraged to wear their ties to the group as political armour are derived from similar thinking, although individual feelings are elevated as paramount in combination with projection of those feelings to outer forces and institutions.

Fulfilment in such a world view depends upon freedom from

the forces of unseen power and oppressive institutions. While I don't deny the importance of collective action and the potential of the psychological sciences being used as a form of cultural imperialism, helping and fostering even the most basic concepts of psychology and how world views can be a way of protecting us from our deeper selves hold significant implications for Muslim groups in particular.

Patients like Jamil are integrated with Australian society and destined to make a fantastic contribution. As he rose up the corporate ladder, he expressed some guilt that he was losing touch with his Muslim heritage. Was he selling out to Western norms, he expressed, a marker perhaps of the challenges that underlie improvement in the Muslim world when worldly success was conflated with subservience to Western norms. But his lack of any appreciation of the foundations of the society he lived in are a cause for concern.

# 2

# CLOSET GAYS

I was raised to despise homosexuals. They were rotten abominations of nature, a misguided lifestyle choice undertaken by those who were consumed by evil influences, most likely the devil in its most accessible form: Western social freedoms. The devil in Islam had the connotation of temptation and its form had its greatest overlap in sexuality, hence the reason why any aspect of female sexuality aroused such passion.

It was a topic that rarely came up in our household. My parents were not particularly religious and did not hold strong views surrounding alternative sexuality. Return visits to my mother's Bangladeshi village were often the only time the topic was broached – for an uncle residing in the mud brick household adjacent to my maternal grandparents displayed the camp, flamboyant behaviours sometimes associated with homosexuality. It was rumoured he was in a relationship with another man in the same village. They were the only gays in the Bangladeshi village.

Sexual relations with the same sex are common however in sexually repressed societies like Bangladesh and other Muslim countries. Early sexual encounters in such regulated communities are more likely to be with close friends of the same sex or even relatives and the vast majority settled into heterosexual relationships later in life.

But the rumours surrounding my uncle turned out to be true and they remained in a long-term relationship, even while one married and had children. They were tolerated but not discussed. Homosexuality was, for the usual minority, something one did and not something one was and provided there was no outward display of any kind that may damage the honour of the family, it was often accepted.

It was in the Sunday school I attended to learn Arabic and read the Koran where more hateful views were communicated. Koranic recounting of the stories of Sodom and the sin of homosexuality being punished by stoning came up not from discussions about sexuality, but from practising our Arabic reading and sifting through the Koranic text.

Such uncomfortable topics coming up on a Sunday afternoon with young teenagers was awfully inconvenient for our Arabic teacher, who attempted to dilute the connotations of the text that, which effectively suggested homosexuality was punishable by death. The teacher was a bearded, middle aged man who spoke incessantly about the injustices handed out to Palestinians, even while he was teaching the Arabic alphabet to teenagers. It was an early lesson of the sheer skills of textual gymnastics that were required to be a Muslim scholar. They forever had to offer reinterpretations of problematic text and to be regularly able to quote contradictory passages to overturn inconvenient proclamations. These varied from permission to hit wives to the sanctioned murder of non-Muslims.

To our teacher's credit, he tried to soften the verse and frame homosexuality much like tax evasion, it was an illegality to be avoided lest one got into trouble with the authorities.

But gay behavior being a betrayal of the natural order was the message in Islamic prophetic passages like "When a man lies with another man, the throne of heaven shakes."

In combination with the rugged masculinity celebrated in Australian boyhood and experienced in the school playground with regular insults of poofter and faggot, it was clear to me that homosexuality was be looked down upon, very much like a disease.

This was, in fact, exactly how my chosen profession, psychiatry, had framed it for decades until it was removed from the classification system, Diagnostic and Statistical Manual in 1973, amid the backdrop of the civil rights movement and greater sexual freedom. Its removal was a good example in how politics helped shape psychiatric diagnoses, given protesters helped overturn the decision making by experts.

Greater exposure to friends and fellow students coming out gay at university helped moderate my views. A friend from high school moved on from the school playground to become the head of Sydney University's gay association, Gloss. I even attended one of their parties in support, and quite enjoyed the attention from the men. I felt a natural connection with their interest in dance and emotional sensitivity, a reprieve from a focus on sculling beer in other university associations.

Not that it helped my Gay-dar. I was consistently the last person amongst my friends to recognize someone as gay. This was particularly embarrassing when I deferred university for a year and travelled around Europe. In Amsterdam I found myself at one of the city's largest gay nightclubs and stumbled on to an entire floor of booths being used for clandestine, and mostly not so clandestine, sexual acts.

On another occasion, while walking in the outer suburbs of Paris, I befriended a cyclist named Jean who offered me directions. My convivial nature and urge to connect after travelling unaccompanied for several months led to further conversation. Jean was an academic at the Sorbonne working on linguistic theory. He was intrigued by my background as a Bangladeshi Australian, spoke of his love for Asia and invited me back to his house for lunch. Sure, he was well dressed, articulate and, in hindsight, perhaps slightly camp but I assumed this had more to do with him being European rather than gay.

A lovely meal of cassoulet and red wine followed, in his apartment not far from the banks of the Seine. I congratulated myself on my growing ability to penetrate the people and culture beyond the tired backpacker trails. Jean offered to make a cup of coffee while suggesting I sit on his white leather couch. Soon afterwards, he sat unusually close to me and turned on gay pornography on the television. How could I not have seen this coming?

After a brief period of shock, I was apologetic. There were no hard feelings. I explained that I was straight and had enjoyed lunch very much. We exchanged details and promised to send letters in the future. Jean said he hoped to travel to Bangladesh one day. I urged him to do so. I left wondering if my desire for home-cooked French food had clouded my judgement.

Years later when I was practising as a doctor and seeing first-hand the challenges of being homosexual, from having partners dying with AIDS to the psychological conflicts inherent in such a challenging identity, I gained a greater empathy for the homosexual experience. I will never forget a young Muslim man in his early twenties who arrived to my western Sydney practice in a state of desperation. His referral letter from his GP was brief, just one line stating that Abdullah was in emotional distress and wanted to consult with a psychiatrist. Dressed in a baseball cap, blue jeans and checked T-shirt, he walked in hesitantly before breaking down into tears, head bowed and resting on his lap.

"I don't want to hurt my family. My mother won't cope," he said, wiping tears from his eyes as I scrambled to get more tissue boxes. I sat with him for almost an hour while he expressed his love for his family and his belief they would never accept his homosexuality.

There was nothing particularly unusual about this upbringing. His father worked as a stonemason before suffering an injury and claiming the disability pension. His mother had been a homemaker all her life, raising seven children. They socialized with extended family and had a close attachment with inhabitants of their former village in Lebanon who all migrated to Australia during the civil war in the 1970s.

Abdullah was one of the youngest children in a large family but he expressed a good relationship with his father, which was another reason why disappointing him was more difficult. Homosexuality has sometimes been framed as a psychic search for a missing father figure, which is why the youngest male children in large families were believed to have a greater vulnerability in past psychological theories, but much of this has since been disproven.

While Abdullah had been in some casual relationships, they were only ever single encounters. He had never been in an intimate relationship despite being twenty-two years old and had kept his sexual orientation a secret. He reluctantly volunteered the story of his last sexual encounter where he met a man through a smartphone application, returned to the man's house and engaged in wild intercourse. He said his actions bordered on violence and the man suffered anal tears. Abdullah apologized but rushed home soon afterwards and head butted the walls in a fit of self-loathing and shame.

His deception was so elaborate that he even bragged to his friends at university, where he was studying engineering, that he picked up girls at nightclubs and had visited brothels. I suspected he was also the most vocal in expressing homophobia. When seen in conjunction with his physical appearance of brimming with muscles he was the picture of faux hyper-masculinity. These were all lies and macho posturing. Perhaps he thought if he acted manly enough, his homosexuality would just go away.

What I found extraordinary was here was a highly educated, clearly intelligent young man who still believed, or at least hoped, that homosexuality could be cured. While engineering was a technically oriented degree and perhaps didn't expose Abdullah to the world of ideas in the humanities, his view of homosexuality was evidence of the power of the traditional cultural beliefs within his community. He was the epitome of the kind of case psychology, and in particular psychoanalysis, aimed to treat – allowing people to exist as individuals outside what were sometimes the prisons of their social context. Freud wrote of his subject matter as "what is most intimate in mental life, everything that a socially independent person must conceal." Abdullah had much to conceal.

"I know the power of tradition and pleasing one's family", I said, trying to sympathise. "My parents wanted me to have an arranged marriage with a girl from Bangladesh." Psychiatrists have different attitudes to self-disclosure, but I found it conducive to a better therapeutic relationship.

"I'm a closet gay Muslim but would prefer to stay inside. I guess I just have to turn the closet into a walk-in-wardrobe," he joked in a rare display of light heartedness during the session. He broke down again soon after.

Abdullah was aware of some past treatments that attempted to cure homosexuality, one of many regrettable phases in the history of psychiatry, illustrated by this passage from *Time Magazine* in February 1965:

> One reason why homosexuals are so rarely cured is that they rarely try treatment. Too many of them believe they are actually happy and satisfied the way there are. Another reason... is that too many psychiatrists are inhibited by the 45 year old pessimism of Freud, who was convinced the condition was discouragingly difficult to treat.

Abdullah asked about electric shock therapy, the only time in my career when a patient actively wished for the treatment. It was one of the more heartbreaking one-off consultations I have ever had with a patient, especially as he left in as much distress as when he arrived, having heard emphatically that there was no cure for being gay. He wanted me to prescribe him tablets like anti-androgens that inhibit testosterone to at least suppress his sexuality but this was unethical. My job was to help Abdullah come to terms with himself, a self that was in opposition with centuries of cultural beliefs embedded in ancestry and religion. His migration to an otherwise sexually liberal country did not change this for him.

I reassured him male homosexuality had a reasonable biological basis, with twin studies showing a thirty per cent concordance, which meant a gay identical twin had a one in three chance of also being gay. This was lower in women suggesting that environmental factors played a greater role. This was my experience in practice where women were more likely to have experienced a traumatic sexual assault and were more likely to "turn gay" later in life, sometimes solely from meeting a particular woman who they felt a strong emotional attraction towards. But this was rarely the case for males, who felt an attraction towards boys as teenagers in the school playground.

I offered to speak to Abdullah's parents to explain the immutability of sexual orientation, but Abdullah was not ready to break their hearts. I also explained that parents, even highly traditional or religious ones, can surprise and that love of one's children diluted pre-existing prejudices, although this was not universal. He could play a critical role in helping to change attitudes within his family and community.

I hoped to establish enough of a relationship that he might return. He had alluded to his sexuality with his family doctor, but in his frank disclosure to me he had exposed himself fully. I felt the privilege of my job in observing people at such times. I hoped Abdullah might consider another resource I had up my sleeve, an interesting group for closet gay patients, introduced by another patient of mine.

As far as closet gays go, Stephen was intriguing. I first met him as a hospital inpatient. A Caucasian, bespectacled man in his forties, he had been transferred from a public hospital after attempting to hang himself in his garage with a self-made noose. It was not a particularly effective attempt for the rope knot loosened almost immediately and he found himself flat on his back on the floor before his wife discovered him and called the police and ambulance.

I remember assessing him late one afternoon as he sat on a bed with a flower filled vase adjacent on a bedside table. He smiled nonchalantly, offering his hand to shake. What was striking was that despite having just attempted suicide soon after his wife threatened to leave him, his behaviour was as if we were meeting at a dinner party or at a work drinks for clients.

"Very sorry to trouble you Dr Ahmed. I know you're very

busy. I hope your practice is going well," he begun, sitting on the edge of the bed with a contained posture, the palms of his hands on his lap.

His day job was working as a salesman, and presenting an image of trouble-free charisma was his bread and butter. It was all he had to fall back on, even during one of his lowest moments.

Stephen was discharged from the public hospital after an overnight stay. Lay people are always amazed when they read people are discharged within a day of making self-harm attempts, but such acts are often made on impulse and there is little a public hospital can do once patients are no longer expressing such thoughts of self-injury.

Stephen's wife had discovered him surfing gay pornography on the internet. Preceding this was a year and a half of erectile dysfunction. His wife stated in the history to the emergency department that her husband had struggled to maintain erections for a long time. While they attempted a handful of counseling sessions and medications like Viagra, progress was limited.

Stephen was cagey with me about the details and said he was "just surfing", adamant he experienced no arousal by the sight of nude men or explicit photos of homosexual acts.

I continued to see him approximately twice a week for three weeks, before he was ready to return home. I placed him on anti-depressants, not because I thought he was depressed but that he seemed highly anxious, often agitated during appointments and complaining of aches and pains in his chest. A little known fact about anti-depressants is that they are more effective for treating anxiety than they are for a depressed mood.

Panic often presents in the form of chest pain, a bane of emergency departments. If health budgets threatened the financial stability of Western economies, a key contributor were the multitudes of people on whom we spend enormous resources to exclude heart disease when they were actually having panic attacks.

What followed over several months of therapy was, initially, going through the motions. As was often the case with many men, there was a matter-of-fact practicality to our meetings, a professional tit for tat. Each session was a business meeting. Stephen would inevitably arrive dressed in a shirt and tie from work and refer to the challenges of the Sydney market. His marriage stayed afloat briefly, but once his mental condition appeared stable his wife wanted a separation. He was adamant that he wanted to stay in the relationship and claimed it had been loving and functional, which seemed at odds to his wife's account of his erectile dysfunction and failed attempts at relationship counselling. If denial was a river in Egypt, my practice made me feel like we were living underwater.

The separation was amicable at first but soon descended into conflict and farce. Mediation failed, lawyers and court loomed and I found myself having to provide progress reports on Stephen's therapy. My notes were regularly subpoenaed, something I was acutely aware of during each consultation, encouraging copious record keeping.

A difficult aspect of being a psychiatrist is the incessant requirement to offer a diagnosis when for the majority of patients it holds a limited relevance. It's a testament to the problematic systems of diagnosis that the profession, notably DSM and its diagnostic offerings such as pre-menstrual dysphoria or oppositional defiant disorder, seemingly medicalise all aspects of human behaviour. In truth, it was merely a pointer at how little we still knew about mental illness.

With Stephen, the therapy was about helping him come to better understand himself, support him through a major loss, and help him integrate the current transition in his life. Success would allow him to be a good father, maintain meaningful relationships and engage in purposeful activity, which for him was working in  sales. But when it came to writing a report, I wrote that he suffered depression, an accessible term that nobody could argue with. I alluded to a likely underlying personality disorder but was wary that it might offer rope to the wife's lawyer in any custody dispute.

During the court proceedings, Stephen arrived more hopeful and optimistic. He had begun dating again through his network in the local church.

"It is a woman," he quickly reassured me with a wry grin. "She is a personal trainer and looks great."

I was not yet sure that he was gay or straight but encouraged him to pursue the potential relationship. From Stephen's reports, the woman from Church was very eager, regularly emailing, texting and wanting him to stay the night. They had several lunches and coffees together before a dinner led to an offer to stay at Cherie's house. I had seen him that week and reduced some of his medications with the view that not only had some of his condition stabilized but that the medications may hamper any sexual response, especially given his history of  failed erections. My wife may find it slightly disturbing that I wondered about whether patients like Stephen had been able to have an erection or not. That weekend was one such occurrence. He had been able to masturbate but when it was time for opening night and the curtains were flung open, would the performance flow?

Alas, it did not – something he expressed deep disappointment about at our next consultation. The event appeared to be a chance to prove to himself that he could still be straight, an indicator of the considerable ambivalence he still experienced about his sexuality. He tried on one more occasion before Stephen let Cherie down with the explanation that he was not ready for a relationship during his painful divorce.

It was also during this time that Stephen spoke about his upbringing. Raised in a strongly religious household, his English father had a considerable temper that was exacerbated by alcohol, usually Scotch whisky. Stephen's only sibling was a younger brother and they were not close. He worried his brother might be taking his ex-wife's side during the divorce.

"I hardly drink because of my father," Stephen said during one consultation while recounting his determination to be a good father to his kids. "He usually smelled of whisky after coming back from the office."

Stephen's father was an accountant running a suburban practice in a leafy suburb of Sydney. The family regularly attended church and Stephen attended a Catholic school.

"How else do you differentiate yourself from your father?" I asked, recognizing there was some ambivalence. There has been such a generational change in the role of fathers that almost all my patients, particularly males, describe wanting to be more emotionally involved in the lives of their children.

"I try not to get angry. He always got angry," Stephen said.

"How do you do that?"

"Well, I just do it. I told myself that I wouldn't get angry like my father."

"How angry did he get?"

"Never violent or anything like that. But I remember him

growling at Mum all the time. When I was a teenager I told myself I wouldn't be like that," he finished.

"How would people know if you were upset or angry?"

"Well…I don't know. I guess they wouldn't."

"It is something apparent in our meetings. I have never seen you particularly distressed outwardly, yet I have you on powerful medications which you are helped by."

Rage was not as culturally sanctioned in Anglo-Saxon cultures especially in comparison to Mediterranean or Arab ones where being too contained communicated disinterest. I had grown up with dramatic displays of emotion, including rage. Arms flailing, voices raised and histrionic performances were all part of showing people you cared or that some kind of need was not being met. But the order so celebrated and perfected by British bureaucracy was sometimes detrimental when applied to the psyche and its encouragement of emotional self-containment.

Coming from a religious background Stephen worried his father would not approve of his divorce, that he might have a need to be angry. He continued to be closely involved in the Church and counted one of the pastors as a confidant.

A few months after he broke off the brief relationship with Cherie I was heartened to hear that he had begun to speak to his pastor about the place of homosexuals in the Church. It was hard not to think of this as an admission of his sexuality but he insisted that he wasn't sure he was gay. He recounted being sexually attracted to his wife in the initial years of his marriage and never being attracted to boys as a teenager. But when I asked what he thought of when he masturbated, he admitted it was fantasies of men.

I wondered why he remained so reluctant to tell me he was gay. It seemed unlikely he would straight out lie to me. It was possible he was responding to me as he did to other authority figures in his life, a bit like the Church or perhaps his father.

It was actually his Church pastor who provided the next impetus. He referred Stephen to a specific counsellor who he thought would suit the situation, namely someone who had experience with closet gays from a Christian background.

Stephen immediately clicked with the new counsellor which aided our consultations also, giving them a greater sense of purpose and direction. His divorce had also been completed and the shared custody arrangements had finally been settled.

Stephen started using the term "same sex attracted". He couldn't yet bring himself to use the term gay, yet it was a major breakthrough. He also seemed reassured by his pastor that he would still be accepted by the Church, which I though was an enlightened interpretation. I doubt a similar response might arise from a mosque cleric.

During this period Abdullah was due to see me again but he failed to attend. I felt compelled to contact him but he brushed off his non-attendance, saying he had another appointment.

Stephen, meanwhile, was going from strength to strength and started attending a group aimed at closet gays. Run by a middle-aged psychologist who came out well into his first marriage, they met once a month in the inner city. I was invited to speak about psychiatric treatments one evening.

I listened attentively to the eight or nine members who attended. They varied in terms of their stages of exiting the closet. A new, very nervous arrival was an Italian man in his forties who expressed guilt at beginning an affair with a gay man. They had met over the web. He expressed great affection for his wife, the mother of his two children, and said he always knew he was gay but felt his traditional, Catholic parents would never accept him.

While other members of the group had progressed to either having admitted the truth to their families or were on the verge, some spoke of their situation for the first time. The relief was visible in their faces. Here was one place where they didn't need to hide. This private group was performing a valuable service. I wished Abdullah could attend, but knew it was unlikely.

Almost all of the men were from some kind of strongly Christian background, usually Catholic. There was one older man from a small country town whose father fought in the Second World War. He was able to come out only when his father had died a few years prior. The theme of not disappointing fathers, as the symbols of authority and tradition, was typical. While psychological theories relating to absent dads were no longer seen as explanatory it was difficult not to see the link in this group. Their homosexuality could be seen as a search for an affection in the arms of a male, affection they felt they never received or feared losing from their fathers. Having said that, if every son who felt neglected or mistreated by their fathers became homosexual, the Sydney Gay and Lesbian Mardi Gras would run for weeks.

I saw Stephen on only one other occasion. We planned for him to reduce his medication to a low dose. He was beaming and admitted he had begun his first gay relationship with a Thai man using a social media platform. He referred to himself as gay and had sat down with his children to explain the situation. His ex-wife was not the slightest bit surprised.

In assessing the effects of any medication side effects, aspects of his sexual performance needed to be raised. With a wry grin, the salesman proclaimed his bliss and glory of experiencing effective erections in the presence of someone he was genuinely attracted to. I thought he might have future problems in regulating anger, but the foundation of his psychic distress had been dealt with.

I emailed Abdullah on another occasion with the details of the group. I hoped he might be able to see a similarity in his situation with the other men who felt trapped in their religious tradition. While Catholicism espoused a greater tolerance of homosexuals than Islam, the teachings were nevertheless unequivocal that homosexuality was against the natural law of the universe.

The situation was even more dire for Muslims, illustrated by the fact that being gay was punishable by death in several Islamic countries. Terrorist attacks in Orlando, Florida, and on the French Riviera have involved Muslim men whose histories suggested the possibility of them being closet homosexuals.

While psychiatry no longer considered the practice of homosexuality as a mental illness, for almost a decade after removing it as a disorder the classification system used the term 'ego-dystonic homosexuality' as a way to describe the psychic distress many gays felt, their physical urges at odds with their idealised self-image. The term seemed apt to me when I saw patients like Abdullah or Stephen. Moreover, its possible contributions to terrorist attacks seemed to be an apt symbol of aspects of Islam itself, an idealised self-image of its former civilizational dominance at stark odds with the modern reality of political and intellectual decline. If the religion was a person, it might also be described as ego-dystonic. By this reckoning, Islamic fundamentalism represented a failure of mourning.

I did eventually hear from Abdullah. He returned my email several weeks later, its contents revealing an outward religiosity and a plan for new relationship adventures.

Assaalaam alaykum brother. Thanks so much for looking out for me Dr Ahmed. I feel a little embarrassed about our meeting many months ago. You'll be pleased to know I have finished my degree and am currently in Lebanon with my new wife. We married here in Beirut a couple of weeks ago. It was a great wedding- 800 people and my family are ecstatic. Inshallah, I hope she will be able to live in Australia soon.

# 3

# FRAGILE NATION

I grew up watching films like *Rambo* and *Platoon* and always imagined that those suffering from post-traumatic stress were ticking time bombs liable to explode with rage at any moment. I pictured sufferers waking to the sounds of helicopters, perhaps with the backing of loud rock music.

I have not endured circumstances I could consider as life threatening. I have watched patients die in front of me, observed drunken, violent assaults and been threatened many times, but the experience of seeing my life flash before my eyes, as many patients describe in such periods, I am not privy to.

During a time I briefly lived in southern Spain, my flatmate and I were walking in the cobblestone streets of the old city of Seville and asked a disheveled man dressed in an overcoat for the time. To our bemusement he slowly pulled a silver revolver from his pocket, showed its contours to us like he was modelling a consumer product, before saying, "*Corre, corre*", which meant "run, run". Run we did. The encounter was too confusing to be considered life threatening, but I did experience dreams replaying the incident for a few days and ruminated on its potential possibilities.

In a particularly bookish, academic version of flashbacks, for a few weeks I dreamt of pictures on a computer screen with the word FAIL in giant capital letters, which is exactly what stared back at me when I failed my specialist examinations for the second time by a paltry one mark. I fell in a heap and questioned my career future, but eventually recovered to pass on my third attempt.

These are normal reactions to stressful events and not indicative of post-traumatic stress disorder. Vivid dreams are a common way we express uncertainty or dread about the future, a clear example of when dreams are an expression of our subconscious. On other occasions dreams can stem from excess, random thoughts spilling out nocturnally, a kind of flatulence of the mind. Memories give us our subjective sense of self. I am in awe of their power when I see patients trapped in the prison a very specific, traumatic memory.

But in my relatively brief career as a psychiatrist I have been amazed by the number of people who walk into my office thinking they might be suffering from PTSD (Post-traumatic stress disorder). Along with bipolar and ADHD (Attention deficit hyperactivity disorder), it is one of the most common diagnoses patients mistakenly think they suffer. PTSD is increasingly a synonym for experiencing adversity, measured subjectively, whereas the original meaning of trauma referred to unexpected, life-threatening circumstances that overwhelmed our coping response.

The steady trickling down of the language of trauma, from initially referring to frontline combatants to now its usage endemic throughout the entirety of civilian life, reflects changing notions of human vulnerability in Western societies. PTSD is now an important cultural narrative to process suffering.

Australian social psychologist Professor Nicholas Haslam refers to this trend as 'concept creep'. He argues that terms like bullying, prejudice, abuse and trauma "now encompass a much broader range of phenomena than before and reflect an ever-increasing sensitivity to harm."

Beyond individual patients I have treated for PTSD, I have been intrigued in recent years as the notion of psychological harm becomes a greater issue in public debates, be it around workplace bullying, same sex marriage or racial discrimination. For example, the Australian Psychological Association supported limiting free speech around the Racial Discrimination Act due to its potential for causing psychological harm to minority groups. One of the key arguments for blocking the plebiscite for same sex marriage was its potential to cause psychological harm to homosexuals. This is a novel application of the John Stuart Mill idea of limiting individual freedom at the point where it causes harm to others. At no stage was this idea ever meant to encompass the notion of psychological harm, but our more "feelings focused" times have altered its application, allowing mental health experts to be used as allies in ideological debates.

I have several patients who are war veterans and have received government benefits for several decades but who did not fight anywhere near the front line of battle. One was an entertainer who became anxious at hearing vivid stories about death and destruction from the soldiers he mixed with. His claim was accepted, legitimising his view that the experience was traumatic and allowed him to consider himself incapable of working at the same level for the rest of his life. The diagnosis became his identity and rendered him psychologically disabled.

Another patient I have consulted for several years in a regional town first arrived stating he had suffered a psychological injury while serving in the navy. I imagined breath-taking tales of battle, perhaps firing cannons or watching missiles batter neighbouring ships. It emerged he was a kitchen hand working in the canteen of one of the battleships and felt unfairly criticised by his boss for the way he prepared the food. He found the boss to be excessively intimidating and suffered panic attacks as a result.

His case could reasonably be considered a work-related injury and, perhaps for a few years, it would be appropriate to support him before he recovered and found alternative work. But when his claim was accepted as a version of post-traumatic stress disorder no different from someone staring death in the face in the frontline infantry, he suddenly had a system of meaning to justify him not working for the next two decades.

When the Department of Veteran Affairs asked me to write a report about his condition and I suggested I couldn't find any, they unfairly recommended he should return to work. My view was that he was no longer employable after being out of the workforce for so many years. You can't give people a way of making sense of their lives for several decades, even if it is mistaken, and then expect to take it away. I fought for him and made sure he could not be taken off the pension, that he was effectively unemployable anyway, despite no longer fulfilling a traditional psychiatric diagnosis.

This steady shift of the notion of trauma into daily life is changing the way we view adversity and making more of us feel less in control of our lives. Two cases highlight this difference between combatants suffering a traumatic syndrome versus civilians acquiring it as an unhealthy way to make sense of their lives when things don't go their way.

Barry entered my office in a whirl of fluorescence, hyperventilation and dirt. His workplace referred him to me under the banner of "veteran affairs" due to his past army service. After a verbal altercation with a fellow worker, he had been placed on his final warning. Wearing blue jeans and a bright vest over a thick, long sleeve shirt, he was the embodiment of Australia's mining economy as he scattered red dirt around my office. Barry worked as a driver of an excavator for a mining site involved in aluminium extraction. He had managed to keep his job for almost eight years, but he informed me early that he was known as someone to steer clear of.

"They say I should have a 'Handle With Care' sign on my forehead," he said.

His face and cheeks had a puffy, red tinge. My eyes drifted towards his hands to assess if there was a tremor typical of alcohol withdrawal – there was not. This was his fourth altercation at work in the past two years and management was considering termination. They had taken all possible measures, from allowing him a repetitive, low stimulation job, giving him extra leeway for breaks, and minimising his interaction with others.

In the late '90s Barry had served in Rwanda for almost eighteen months as a private on a peacekeeping mission, during what has been widely reported as one of the worst genocides of the twentieth century. After his return, he struggled to function in any of the five different roles he was assigned to in the defence forces, from paperwork to answering phone calls to assisting with maintenance.

When I asked him why he stopped working for the army he shook his head and said, "I just couldn't do it. It was like I was demented or something." But it wasn't a medical discharge, just a voluntary one.

Jai was a thin, young man born in the South Indian city of Madras. He entered my western Sydney rooms grabbing at his neck brace with one hand and carrying a pile of documents in the other. His wife walked beside him, opening doors and organising the seating.

Jai looked forlorn. He was barely audible when he began his story, shuffling through his documents and fiddling with his phone as he spoke.

"I was bullied, you know, terribly," he said, reaching once more towards his neck. "It was racial abuse."

Jai put his smartphone on to the desk separating us, scrolled through his text messages before turning the phone towards me so I could read them.

The first text Jai showed me said, "You smell a bit like curry today. I bet your wife's a good cook."

Another read, "You've got a pretty good job, don't ya...all the Indians I know are cleaners or in servos."

He scrolled down to a final text, "I love that new flat top you got. Ha. It's a shocker, mate. You gotta get some fashion advice."

Rather than detailing the story, Jai then drew several business cards from his selection of documents. One stated that he was the team leader at a data processing section of a New Zealand energy company.

"I was very senior there," he said.

Next he showed me a picture of him receiving an award for community contribution, also during his time in New Zealand.

"They told me that Australians were a bit rough, but I have never been treated so badly," said Jai in reference to his work colleague, before turning to his wife who was holding back tears. "He has taken my life."

Jai had migrated from New Zealand where he, his wife and two children had lived for five years. He worked in an office role and had trained in accounting back in India. His first job in Australia was for an insurance call centre. He had not worked for several months and was filing a legal suit for workplace bullying.

"Tell me about the neck?" I asked, confused about the brace.

"Car accident. Whiplash," Jai informed me, pulling out a letter from a hospital in Bangalore.

He was a passenger in a car involved in an accident, which left him with neck stiffness. When nothing is revealed from imaging tests such as X-rays and CT scans, ongoing neck pain is classified as whiplash. Jai suffered the injury in the weeks after taking sick leave from his job, during which he visited relatives in India.

He continued to wear a neck brace for months afterwards and described tightness and pain emanating from the back of his shoulders to the back of his head. I immediately considered the pain to be more likely an expression of anxiety, rooted in his feeling of humiliation, but did not press him so early in our interactions. Like all psychological symptoms, his pain had a meaning and not acknowledging it was a recipe for disaster.

Jai described regular nightmares where he walked alone in an empty office unable to find his desk. He didn't have flashbacks of his alleged assailant, the man who sat in the adjacent booth in his office, but noted his headaches worsened whenever he would read the text messages on his phone.

Like many influential ideas during the twentieth century, from management consulting to the internet, knowledge surrounding psychological breakdown arose through the army and the experience of soldiers in combat. War provides an exaggerated version of the human experience. It gives us unique insights into the borders of our humanity.

According to the British military psychiatrist Professor Simon Wessely, knowledge surrounding the symptoms of psychological breakdown in combat has been well known for over a century and perfected even more so through the World Wars. It had different names such as 'shell shock' or 'war neurosis'. In the mid-twentieth century Western asylums were full of ex-servicemen with such syndromes. In a 2005 paper for the *British Journal of Psychiatry* Wessely writes:

> For the first half of the 20th century it was assumed that if you broke down in battle, and the cause was indeed the stress of war, then your illness would be short-lived – and if it was not, then the cause of your ill health was not really the war at all, but events before you went to war…if you broke down and never recovered, then the real cause was not the war, but either your genetic inheritance or your upbringing. The war was merely the trigger.

The Vietnam War transformed the way we viewed trauma, but this transformation was driven more by politics than any new physiological discoveries. By the 1970s the Vietnam veteran developed into a serious political liability – alienated by society and disturbed by horrible nightmares from the war experience, they were seen as something of a social time bomb. To explain this trend psychiatrists introduced an entirely new term into the diagnostic language- the condition of post-traumatic stress disorder.

So what was original about the new diagnosis? That large numbers of mentally ill soldiers might emerge from war was not news: established thinking at the time taught that if you experienced long-term psychiatric complications then the war experience was the trigger and not the real cause.

But in the context of the simmering public outrage at an unpopular conflict, the architects of PTSD did not accept the established view. They believed with good intentions that the war was undoubtedly to blame.

One of the first descriptions of the syndrome was written by psychoanalyst Dr Chaim Shatan and published in *The New*

*York Times* in 1972. His argument was that Vietnam veterans felt upset because they had been 'deceived, used and betrayed' by a combination of the military, the government and society at large. Shatan alluded to the veteran's rage but did not suggest this was a particular reaction to life-threatening battlefield encounters. He described it as what "follows naturally from the awareness of being duped and manipulated".

As anthropologist Ethan Watters writes about the syndrome, "it was the moral ambiguity of the Vietnam War and the deceitfulness of the US government and military, not the trauma of battle, that damaged the psyche of the soldier".

But tuning in to the political currents of the time, the diagnosis caught on with tremendous success and attracted other clinicians wanting to extend the concept to other horrors, varying from natural disasters to fire and motor vehicle accidents. What changed was that the cause of PTSD was the 'T' – the trauma. The attraction and danger lay in its clean simplicity. Most psychiatric diagnoses did not implicate a cause, but here was one with a designated origin: adult trauma.

The messy business of dissecting heredity and upbringing could be replaced with the purity of the experience of war. As outlined by war historian Eric Dean's book *Shook Over Hell*, there was no new physiology or science to support the claim, only the new politics. The diagnosis was designed to shift the focus from the soldier's background and psyche to the fundamentally traumatic characteristic of war.

My patient Barry tells me about the first few weeks of returning home to his regional town. One day he walked with his daughter to the main street with the aim of getting a haircut. He remembered feeling exposed, having been used to military colleagues covering him as he scoured the streets for threats and monitored roofs and windows for snipers. While he knew rationally that it was not Rwanda, the primitive recesses of his mind did not differentiate.

"I ran out of the barber's with shaving cream all over me," he said, breaking down in tears. "I just thought it would get better." A combination of noises outside the shop – a dog's bark, the loud exhaust of an accelerating car – had triggered an upsurge of adrenalin in Barry that completely overwhelmed him.

The symptoms of a traumatic syndrome are classed in three categories. One is the re-experiencing phenomenon in the form of nightmares or flashbacks. Another is avoidance behaviours of anything that might remind the patient of the traumatic event – for example, survivors of serious car accidents may not be able to drive or even sit in a car for months. The final category is what is known as hypervigilance, where the mind is in a constant state of awareness, scanning the environment for potential threats thereby creating a physiological charge, often making the person appear on edge or highly irritable.

Jai suffered the same symptoms, even though his exposure could not be considered life threatening. His dreams were not true flashbacks. Rather, they were symbolic of his loss of identity and psychic disruption. The images of the text messages from his colleague would play over and over in his mind. He would stare at the business cards from his previous managerial roles to help remind him of better days. He was not faking it, but his work identity was so central to his self-image that any disruption to it was intolerable.

My focus for Jai was to help him see that his physical pain may have been a more acceptable, face-saving way to cope with his sense of humiliation. I wanted to help him realise the pain was a psychological expression rather than something that could be treated with more and more painkillers. Studies show clearly that successfully dealing with trauma depends upon the meaning sufferers attached to the experience and whether they felt they had control over their symptoms and lives. The longer Jai blamed his employer entirely for his symptoms and didn't consider the contribution of his personality and the event's connection with his self-image, the less likely he was to recover.

Barry self-medicated his symptoms away for years, drinking up to fifteen beers a day after coming home from work. His wife suspected there was a serious problem but did not know what to do, and so she focused her life on their young daughters.

"Our marriage was just going through the motions," said Barry, reflecting on his lost years. His ability to manage in his routine, a relatively menial mining job, for all its benefits, probably delayed him receiving treatment.

I called Dr Lavinia Schmidtman, the medical director of St John of God Hospital in Richmond, New South Wales, and head of one of the largest trauma programs in Australia. She said that despite the changes in thinking within the medical fraternity, the Australian Defence Forces and the police, accelerated by the Dunt Review into mental health and the Defence Forces in 2009, have only started taking PTSD seriously in recent years.

Dr Schmidtman estimates that only in the last six or seven years have there been major transformations in how the disorder is treated and monitored within both the police and army. She mentions the deployments of psychologists in the field, regular monitoring of personnel after exposure to combat or traumatic events, and involvement of rehabilitation coordinators to help affected workers return to frontline duties.

Spokespersons from NSW Police and the ADF state that regular, structured programs had been in place since 2000 for the police and

2002 for military personnel, in response to comprehensive reviews into the mental health management of their employees. The focus is on psychological wellbeing in general and neither organisation took responsibility for specialised treatment.

Professor Maureen Dollard is one of Australia's foremost experts on stress and the workplace. In an interview with me she said that psychological risks were not taken seriously in the workplace up until about ten years ago. The focus used to be on mitigating the types of personalities that might make complaints about colleagues or managers, whereas there was now a greater shift in recognising workplaces as a possible contributor to psycho-social risk.

"There is now more of an accepted belief that anybody could be worn down within difficult environments," she said, noting that it reflected similar changes in thinking about psychological trauma.

This view is central to changes in our relationship to adversity and our attitudes towards human frailty. Arguably, Western conceptions of the 'self' have changed from viewing the human being as fundamentally resilient to formulations that view people as innately fragile. It is noticeable that patients like Jai, despite coming from cultures that do not share this outlook, rapidly absorb it as a way to make sense of their suffering.

Professor Dollard also cited the greater tensions between productivity and profit versus the welfare of the workers. She said that work had become the pre-eminent marker of identity and social status, for both women and men, and this exacerbated psychological risks. Furthermore, a service economy depended more heavily upon the human resources, especially the highly skilled variety, making the management of workplace stress and conflict a managerial imperative of the highest order.

The example of Jai illustrates how this greater reliance on work as the primary marker of modern identity, in combination with a loosening of the notions of trauma has precipitated a rapidly burgeoning field of psychological risk in the workplace and society at large. The trauma that Jai was exposed to was of a much smaller magnitude than that of Barry, but his coping resources were nevertheless overwhelmed, resulting in similar symptoms. He was also from a culture that had strong stratifications in class and caste. He had already experienced a significant drop in such status through migration, as most immigrants do, and the humiliation he felt from what others might regard as relatively trivial office banter was a blow too many.

How realistic is it then to attribute the cause to the T, namely the trauma.

The costs of our growing emphasis on human vulnerability are astronomical and rising. According to the Workplace Trauma Project Team at Griffith University, the financial cost of trauma and its manifestations to business is between $6 and $13 billion per year and can include decreased productivity, increased absenteeism, staff turnover and poor morale. The average cost of a bullying claim is $41,500.

Within the police there has been a huge blowout in disability claims relating to mental illness, right across Australia. There are similar trends across the Western world. NSW taxpayers have paid more than $100 million since 2005 to settle them, according to statistics compiled by the NSW government. There has been a 300 per cent increase in mental health cases.

The newfound focus on PTSD has reached a level where the Victorian Police Union, in combination with the state's paramedics, are attempting to lobby the government for further changes to legislation. They are arguing for new laws to ensure all cases of

PTSD are automatically accepted as being caused by their work in either police or the ambulance services, which they argue should be accepted as innately traumatic. This is a stunning example of how the concept of psychological trauma has filtered from the frontline of war to civilian life in the emergency services.

While the experience of trauma may not always result in PTSD, it was often the trigger to claims involving other diagnoses such as depression or anxiety disorders. Work-related psychological disputes are the most expensive form of disability and compensation claims, as they involve lengthy periods of absence from work.

Barry and Jai are examples of the effects of trauma and their relationship with the workplace, and also of how military concepts of trauma have now taken on new meanings within the civilian sphere.

As further outlined by Professor Wessely, the boundaries of psychiatric injury have since widened in barely a few decades. In its initial formulation PTSD could be diagnosed only after situations that had genuinely threatened life and limb. This has expanded to include situations in which people felt in danger, even when this was not at all the case. It has shifted to virtually any adverse experience, from seeing a distressing image on television, receiving a serious health diagnosis to even normal experiences such as giving birth.

The diagnostic label of PTSD has become a synonym for all distress, and shifted from its initial rigorous formulation in the military context to a looser one for civilians. The police are a good marker of societal concepts of trauma for they are a middle ground between the military and civilians.

Dr Doron Samuell, a forensic psychiatrist and strategic adviser to several major insurance companies, believes that, 'Workers are more entitled now. There is almost an expectation among many that there will be no negative feedback or adversity.'

'What has changed is that workers attribute the cause to the workplace and their colleagues, rather than their own coping mechanisms.'

This is a reflection of broader social changes around the primacy of feelings. People ascribe an authenticity in the feelings they experience and are more likely to project difficult or intolerable ones to their external environment. The problem is that when patients become utterly fixated on the sense of injustice and desire for bureaucratic or legal revenge, they struggle to move on with their lives. The most affected are those who have too narrow a view of themselves defined by their work and a rigid, black and white sense of the meaning of justice. This is common in jobs where patients carry a stronger sense of implementing social justice, such as the helping professions of teaching or nursing.

Dr Samuell warns that trauma and its association with bullying has the potential to become an almighty headache for employers since Fair Work changed the law in 2013, whereby there is no longer a requirement for a psychiatric diagnosis after allegations of bullying, something that elevates the subjective experience as an automatic truth.

Professor Dollard said employers had to make a greater emphasis on people managers when considering promotion, sometimes ahead of technical abilities. 'The financial risk of poor people skills is greater than it has ever been.'

I saw Barry one more time before he agreed to try a comprehensive trauma program in Sydney. His nightmares of machete-cut bodies returned with a vengeance as soon as he started reducing his alcohol intake. His wife accompanied him to the appointment and broke down in tears in the consultation room, saying she had given up on their marriage long ago. She didn't think there was any hope.

As he made progress in treatment, he was better able to integrate his experience and incorporate what is known as traumatic growth. Most traumatic experiences do not result in a psychiatric syndrome, but we as a society and particularly the burgeoning, therapeutic complex have become acutely sensitive to its inevitability. What is more likely is that people experience a psychological and spiritual growth, particularly if they are able to ascribe an acceptable meaning to the incident or event. It is difficult for experts like me to predict who will recover when so many of the factors are non-medical, such as Barry's own expectations for improvement, the availability of social supports, and the intimate meaning he makes of his distress.

In Barry's case, a challenge that was common for many veterans since the Vietnam War was that they didn't always return as heroes to their communities or countries. Nor were the wars they were involved in associated with a larger narrative for the story of their countries.

A similar process can occur among the large numbers of police and emergency workers now falling under the PTSD banner. For many, the job does not work how they may have wanted. They experience a conflict with a colleague or fail in a promotion and the notion of a traumatic syndrome is a system of meaning that allows them to make sense of their feeling of loss. Much like the original formulation of PTSD after the Vietnam War, they feel duped by their employer and society but begin to ascribe their sense of feeling wronged to past traumas they experienced in their work. Our memories of past events are strongly affected by current events and mental state.

The notion of PTSD is arguably a cultural product primarily

tied to the modern West's notions of human vulnerability, as argued by Canadian anthropologist Allan Young in his book *The Harmony of Illusions: Inventing Post-Traumatic Stress Disorder*. Professor Young argues it is as much a product of the legal profession as the psychiatric one and linked to a host of cultural currents varying from the suffering of Holocaust survivors, the growth in refugees post-war and the rise of identity politics.

Its cultural success coincides with the decline in other systems of meaning, such as religion. The psychological sciences have taken precedence to help encounter suffering and death. It is usually in crisis through a major loss or trauma that we are shaken enough to question how we ascribe purpose to our lives, and the formulation of PTSD has filled this gap for many. Unfortunately psychiatric diagnoses are often cold comfort and do not easily replace the wider moral and spiritual systems what we have lost.

Jai arrived at his third appointment with a set of forms applying for support with regards to a total and permanent disablement claim, which is defined as having less than a 50 per cent chance of returning to his pre-injury work. After receiving legal advice he wanted compensation for his experience of bullying and didn't think he could return to work.

I found myself in the awkward but typical position of wanting to maintain rapport within the therapeutic relationship, but not wanting to encourage a victim mentality that would delay his recovery. He had at least stopped wearing his neck brace. I suggested he postpone his application until he had further engaged with treatment.

He was polite through the appointment, nodding and grabbing his neck simultaneously. When I asked him about future aspirations, he once again produced his old business cards with their professional titles. As he walked out of the session, he gave me a protracted, exaggerated thank you, the meaning of which I was familiar with.

Jai has not returned since. While it is possible he re-engaged elsewhere and has made progress, I see patients like Jai as those with whom I have failed to instil a sense of individual agency, a kind of defeat to the social and legal institutional incentives embedded in the outside world.

# 4

# ON PURITY

There was a time when I wondered what my true self might be. So, like many students, I took a year off from university to travel, at least partially in the hope I may find myself – a secular pilgrimage to the Mecca of uncovering of my perceived identity, though I had no idea what that might mean.

I found booze, unliveable youth hostels and an inordinate number of historical monuments but, alas, my true self was not hidden in the backstreets of Amsterdam's red light district or exhibited on the walls of the Louvre. Travelling alone for long periods did improve my levels of introspection and the capacity to reflect, which was more valuable than the mysterious allure of self-discovery.

I sensed I was closer to some authentic version of myself when I travelled with my family to visit my parent's village. I enjoyed seeing relatives who had similar facial features, some who had a similar sounding voice. It was clear I had strong roots in this region of Bangladesh adjacent to the Indian border, a place that was strongly homogenous ethnically, but had still enjoyed migration and conquest from Persians, Indo-Aryans and the British.

But while I enjoyed the role play of wearing a singlet, a cloth around my waist called a lungi and working briefly in the rice paddies, it was a privileged travel exercise in trying on the shoes of the poor before returning to a five star hotel. Despite my genetic proximity to my relatives, I had more in common with the Greek mechanic working a block from my house in Sydney.

In my search I left being a doctor to pursue a career in journalism. It lasted only a year and was more of an itch to be scratched, but the exercise taught me that fulfilment was not to be found in what was often a mythical perception of an ideal career, a job that might reflect an authentic self. I enjoyed the storytelling and broad subject matter that journalism offered, but the instant gratification of helping distressed patients that medicine allowed was difficult to match. I have since been able to integrate my interests in storytelling and communication within my work as a psychiatrist.

It is a constant challenge to avoid defining myself too narrowly through the category of my career and achievements, or lack thereof, and recognise the full breadth of my identity as a father, husband, son and friend. This is advice I am forever giving to my patients who view themselves too one-dimensionally through their job. But like so many doctors, it is not always easy to practice what I preach.

This search for self can be easily mocked. The satirical website 'The Onion' had a story titled "Search for Self Called Off After 38 Years", where a fictional character travels extensively, attends health retreats, signs up for multiple creative courses and attempts career changes, not unlike myself, but ends with this advice:

> Trust me — there's nothing out there for you to find. You're wasting your life. The sooner you realize you have no self to discover, the sooner you can get on with what's truly important: celebrity magazines, snack foods, and Internet porn.

While for health reasons I actively limit snack foods, have no interest in celebrity magazines and am too easily caught if surfing internet pornography to participate in it, the various experiences of extended travel and career change gave me an insight into how we live in a cultural tradition in which the significance of our lives is so tightly bound up with self-fulfilment.

There is a complex relationship between self-fulfilment and the notion of authenticity, an idea that we each have some kind of way of living that is uniquely ours. This urge receives much needed dilution after we marry and children arrive, when the needs of our progeny take precedence. Alternatively, the project of self-fulfilment is merely projected upon the children.

But the idea of an authentic self is not a time honoured ideal. Canadian philosopher Charles Taylor, author of a book called *The Ethics of Authenticity*, argues that it emerged only in the late eighteenth century. The idea was that we each have a moral sense and a feeling for what might be right. This moral sense was not considered merely a matter of calculation but was anchored in our feelings. Our inner feelings were considered a link with God and what was innately good. Taylor argues that that ideal of authenticity comes from a corruption of this belief in an intuitive sense of morality or of some kind of conscience that guides us linked to feeling.

The physician and author Carl Elliot writes in his book *Better Than Well* that: "The idea of conscience as a moral guide, the concept of self-fulfillment, our right to pursue our vision of the good life, the notion of psychotherapy uncovering an inner truth buried deep within the unconscious – all these are part of the way in which authenticity has become a crucial part of modern identity."

This focus on the moral significance of the individual resonated with Enlightenment ideas arising from the European revolutions that separated reason from God. This change was necessary before we could see ourselves as rational individuals able to exercise decisions, the basis for which is the cornerstone of the modern State. But the focus on feelings has steadily acquired an alternative direction.

By the middle of the twentieth century, American psychoanalyst Rollo May writes, 'The chief problem of people in the middle decade of the twentieth century is emptiness.' According to May, people felt empty because they didn't know whether their inner lives were truly theirs or not. He believed the source of this failure was not being adequately knowledgeable about one's feelings. It followed that if you were not in touch with your feelings, you could not live a truly meaningful life.

I observe this search for authenticity in a wide variety of patients, from the staunchly religious Muslim channelling his sense of identity through outer markers of religiosity to the vegan hipster attempting to regain a connection with nature. Many modern movements from religious revivalism to paleo diets are rooted in a quest for authenticity, in combat with a secular civic life that can feel bereft of any vision of a transcendent purpose.

The young Muslim living in the West searches for authenticity in attempting to separate what aspects of his religion are stained by local cultural customs, such as those inherited from Hindu traditions in India, versus what was the original practice in sixth century Arabia. This search acquires a new meaning to those living in the West for it is a unique phase where Muslims are living a de-territorialised zone, their practice of Islam is not linked with local customs and culture but being forged anew. An example of this is when my mother and other Muslim women are chided for wearing saris at Friday prayer in a mosque, an event that led to us walking out on one occasion. A similar clash is occurring in

Muslim countries where a local, gentler Islam might clash with stricter, Arabised versions sold as purer and more authentic.

I have struggled to empathise with the lust to connect to nature that I see in many patients and well-off friends. Just as there are patients who believe medications will solve their problems and have little desire to engage in greater self-reflection, there are a growing number of patients who are staunchly opposed to any pharmaceutical tablets believing medication will corrupt their body. The word they mostly use is 'toxic', that the body was never made to process such laboratory designed monstrosities.

Their fears overlap with their views of what constitutes the authentic and a belief that the closer something is to being natural, the more beneficial it may be. The naturalist Wendell Berry argues that the more artificial a human environment becomes, the more the word 'natural' becomes a term of value. The word implies a lack of stain from human limitations, a state where things are engineered wholly by nature, intelligent design or a deity.

I spent my early years in Bangladesh, living in a shared housing estate, my parents, some relatives and myself all sharing two rooms. I have no memory of hardship. It was a free-range existence roaming and playing with other children, of which there were many in the most densely populated country in the world. My first, most powerful memory had a direct overlap with nature and disease. One of the kids I used to play with, a stocky boy called Rojon, had fallen on a metal spike. I was not with him at the time, but remember him complaining about stepping on a rock.

Days later he was rushed to hospital and by nightfall he had died. I was dumbfounded and held tightly in a room by a relative to avoid seeing the corpse, brought back by the father for rapid burial as is Islamic custom. I learnt later that he died of something called tetanus, a germ that penetrated through the screw that lodged in his foot.

In combination with the regular floods that occurred in Bangladesh, I had no illusions that nature was innately benevolent. But my fears were moderated by a childhood that was inextricably linked to the outdoors and no shortage of dirt. There were sprawling slums adjacent to our home in Bangladesh and no official rubbish service. The streets were piled high with foodstuffs, plastic, the smell of urine...you name it. I know this sounds disgusting but it did make the relationship with dirt and mess more relaxed. And this different relationship to the natural world and a greater ease with dirt is perhaps why Asian restaurants are often considered deficient in hygiene practices. The word germ is defined as an organism that can cause disease or can be a part of the body capable of building tissue. It can bring both illness and growth and is derived from a word meaning seed.

I think my ease with dirt was reinforced when we moved to Australia, when freckled, pale-skinned locals were often the ones flushed with allergies and asthma. They were also the most protected, their mothers washing all the time and their bodies entirely covered with clothes and sunscreen. This was partly a function of the Celtic complexion being poorly suited to the climate, but I have always felt my early exposure to the teeming infestation of germs that a Bangladeshi childhood demanded was a source of protection, a kind of heightened immunity. I am not proposing we live in squalor, but adopt a relaxed attitude away from our anti-bacterial soap and perpetual washing. My attitudes continue to cause tension with my wife whenever I lick the spoon while stirring meals.

I have a patient who has taught me a great deal about the beliefs underlying the attraction to alternative medicine and how it can be futile to attack them. His ideas come from the same source as religion and can be an attempt to find something transcendent as old rules and structures crumble. This can apply at both a personal and collective level.

For Angelo, his retreat into alternative foods and medicine occurred as his business started to fail. He is a Filipino man in his fifties, lean and dressed neatly in a sweater and jeans. He didn't present for my services of his own accord, but because his income protection insurance was confused about his lack of recovery and whether some of Angelo's preferred methods of treatment, such as flying to a retreat in California or engaging in a deep breathing course in Byron Bay, were legitimate.

There was always a despondency about Angelo, a sense he was in a struggle for his soul. Like most mental health presentations, they were ultimately about redefining purpose and meaning, usually in the face of crisis or great loss. For Angelo, his problems began soon after the financial crisis of 2007. Prior to that, despite having only a high school education from the Philippines, he was tremendously successful earning hundreds of thousands of dollars in accounting. He was particularly successful in the large Filipino community in western Sydney, but his business expanded beyond that area. His self-image was strongly tied to his financial success and he struggled to cope with the destruction that the financial upheaval wrought. He took what was systemic to the economy very personally.

"I had too much stress, doctor," Angelo said. "I only had time to eat two minute noodles in my five minute breaks." He carried with him his own personal statement consisting of five pages of typed notes. He held his palm to his forehead and said he could never cover all his difficulties in one or two interviews.

Angelo was becoming anxious as his business began to decline, especially as the government enacted laws to strengthen regulations around the accounting industry. He suffered terrible headaches and said his mind began to race. His wife and two daughters tried to be supportive, but Angelo was convinced his problems lay in his diet and lifestyle. He tried seeing a psychologist and was placed on anti-depressants by his family doctor, but he claimed they didn't help.

"Food can cure everything. You don't cure with drugs; food and nature is our medicine. I was such a bad person with food," Angelo said, holding back tears.

He interpreted the failure of his business as a kind of cosmic payback for his sin of not eating appropriately healthy food and failing to adequately engage with nature. Despite claiming insurance for depression, he went to great lengths each day preparing his meals, boiling his vegetables and lining up his vitamins and supplements. His naturopath diagnosed him with a biochemical imbalance known as pyrrole disorder, a syndrome that arose in the 1970s describing a combination of lethargy and aches and pains. The diagnosis has been disproven, but reappears as an entity in alternative medicine circles.

Angelo also joined his bushwalking group each week and conducted his breathing exercises with extra gusto while on the nature trails.

His activities caused a considerable strain within his family. He was no longer intimate with his wife. His daughters were adults and focused on their university studies. Angelo was always socially awkward and utterly devoted to being a financial planner, sending a portion of his income to his extended family living in the Philippines. I sensed his immediate family had given up on him recovering and allowed him to conduct his rituals and routines.

When faced with patients like Angelo, it is difficult to hide my frustration. Here was a patient destroying his life for no good reason other than his resolute determination to hold on to misguided beliefs. I knew what would help him. He needed some low dose medication, some psychological therapy to understand the automatic thoughts that led to his anxiety and a greater flexibility in his self-image. Angelo's challenge was to integrate the loss of either no longer being a wealthy accountant or accept being a not so successful accountant in the latter stages of his working life. Food and nature had nothing to do with it.

His beliefs were the only thing holding him together. Here was his fragmented and fractured attempt to assert himself in the face of the intolerable loss of his career and work identity. I had no chance of helping him if I challenged his fundamental beliefs, much like if I argued against a devout Christian or Muslim for their belief in God. I had to work with them and not against.

There were considerable challenges. Even devout Christians or Muslims did not necessarily view my treatments as fundamentally opposed to their worldview. It was possible for them to combine a moral, religious conception of the human being with a biological and psychological one. Where the problem lay was a lack of trust in traditional authority, be it religious, medical or political. Angelo barely consumed any traditional media, believing it to be too biased. He preferred satellite television from overseas, mainly from the Philippines and a newsletter that his naturopath recommended consisting of lifestyle advice.

Angelo was from a devoutly Catholic background, as was the norm for most Filipinos. When I asked him about his family, he said he had a falling out with his mother after marrying a woman against her wishes. They had mended their relationship but it was never the same. I wondered whether his strict beliefs around food and alternative therapies were a pining for lost maternal bonds, the religious, transcendent overtones a link with a strongly religious childhood. They may also have been symbolic of a protest.

I spent several sessions focusing on building trust between us, allowing him to vent his shame and guilt arising from his business failure. I tried to involve his family, but he was resistant to the idea. He said he didn't want to bother them with his problems, but I suspected he did not want to face what his wife and children really thought about his ascetic withdrawal. He had constructed an elaborate system of denial through organic food and health food supplements.

His situation could only occur in wealthy countries like Australia, where insurance was paying him to remain unemployed and conduct an alternative lifestyle. Angelo did technically tick the boxes for depression, given he was socially withdrawn, had strained family relationships, lacked motivation to work and often suffered disrupted sleep. For this reason, his family doctor regularly filled out the necessary forms for Angelo to obtain income protection every few months. But he was also able to maintain a highly structured daily routine, planned meticulously. What incentive did he have to change?

Not a great deal, I soon discovered. He politely accepted my prescriptions for medication and my extensive explanations that such small doses were unlikely to cause side effects and were not 'toxic' in any way. But he never commenced my suggested treatments, continuing his daily routine instead. Our therapeutic relationship was improving however, and I noticed he was more jovial at times, less focused on his symptoms and guilt surrounding his diet. But there was no other change in his outlook.

For some of my patients from strict Muslim or Pentecostal Christian backgrounds, sometimes their imam or pastor became involved in their treatments. Their involvement helped to link the moral, spiritual side with what felt like dry, technical treatments from the cold efficiency of modern medicine. This kind of practice is known as integrated or culturally sensitive treatment. Involving an Aboriginal liaison officer with indigenous patients is similar. But what to do with a patient like Angelo? Should I have attempted to involve his naturopath or perhaps a lifestyle chef, a nod to the quasi-religious authority they now held?

Orthorexia is a relatively new term in the health lexicon, but one that applies to an increasing number of people. It refers to people who are fixated on eating correctly in accordance to a strict and punitive understanding of what's healthy to eat as well as what must be strongly avoided. In the book The Wellness Syndrome, authors Carl Cederstrom and Andre Spicer argue this behaviour has its roots in 'biomorality', which they define as "the moral demand to be happy and healthy".

The worldview has strong overlaps with humanistic psychology and the rise of positive thinking – that you can will your way to worldly success and failure is a function of mindset. Despite its soft outward glow, this outlook is deeply conservative and libertarian in its outlook. Applied to physical health, the body becomes its own truth system and encourages a kind of withdrawal into passive nihilism. But when it's applied on a more collective level, for example as some public health movements wanting to ban junk food, or happiness experts employed by corporations, the entire philosophy of demanding so-called "wellness" starts looking like tyrannical ideology.

The notion of wellness began in line with the movements of positive psychology, which had a perfectly reasonable aim of focusing on health prevention as opposed to treating established or burgeoning illness. The website of Complementary Medicines Australia states, "the true strength of naturopathy lies in its underlying philosophy which sees the client as a complete being and the body as a complete system". The statement has all the hallmarks of the authenticity paradigm, a belief that there was some kind of essence not objectively measurable.

For the most part, alternative therapies and diets such as paleo are harmless. According to the National Institute of Complementary Medicine, two-thirds of Australians use complementary medicines every year and spend almost four times as much when compared to pharmaceuticals. Meanwhile, any doctor will tell you that vitamins and supplements are virtually useless in all but the most malnourished or specifically ill people in Western societies, but consumers keep voting with their wallets. The rise of such feelings-based treatments are leading to some major Australian success stories in business. Companies like Blackmores enjoy multi-billion dollar sales in China. I suspect executives at such companies are well aware that their product offers little but placebo treatments, but perhaps the gap lies in modern medicine's failure to understand the power of the placebo.

I visited a naturopath once, in a kind of undercover, spy mission. I didn't reveal myself to be a medical doctor and said I worked as an accountant but had interests in Ayurvedic medicine because of my ethnic background. The naturopath was pleased. I told him that I was suffering a vague lethargy where I didn't always want to get out of bed and felt some mild anxiety in social situations. I said it had been going on for months and didn't seem to be getting better.

He took a lengthy history much like a doctor would and then felt my pulse. I looked around his lemon-scented office and was impressed by the posters of the body, brain and scientific-looking paraphernalia. But once the interview was completed, he pulled out a device and asked to take a couple of pricks of blood. I had worked in a pathology laboratory and not once processed tests referred from a naturopath. He planned to send my blood to look at the red blood cells and examine it for acid. I had heard about live blood cell analysis and knew it to have no scientific basis. The naturopath then suggested I try some supplements. I didn't return and suspect he would have diagnosed me with pyrrole disorder, much like my patient Angelo.

On leaving the naturopath, however, I actually felt quite good. I had enjoyed speaking to him for almost an hour. The appointment began as an undercover, stealth exercise, but by the end of it I just spoke about my personal life away from my career, my interests and my aspirations. The office had a nice ambience too.

There is not a great deal to be gained by bashing alternative health practitioners or purveyors of virtuous food. It is filling some kind of gap. I was impressed at the sheer amount of time I was able to spend with a naturopath. Many of my patients complain how quickly they are churned through a general practice, which are now mostly corporatised. In the past the average person may have sought wisdom and relief for their woes either through the medical profession or perhaps their priest. But doctors are now seen as distracted and too technically oriented, focused on tests and a checklist of symptoms. Meanwhile organised religion is seen as antiquated and irrelevant for large sections of the community. Alternative medicine fills this gap. It's a middle ground between religion and science, which suits the expanding group of the population who see themselves as spiritual but not religious.

What I found interesting about seeing the naturopath was how he had co-opted many of the rituals of traditional medicine. He took a long and detailed history, used a needle to take blood and suggested I buy some pills. But when the idea of me having a certain energy that he, not a medical practitioner or priest, had the power to manipulate, the encounter veered into the supernatural.

The claims of the alternative health sector are not testable, making their powers of explanation enormous and also leaving consumers thinking their problems have a spiritual significance. Its popularity coincides with a time in health when problems of chronic disease dominate and the focus is upon improving function and not cure. This can be dissatisfying for many patients.

American essayist Eula Biss writes in her book On Immunity that acting in a natural way is linked to fears about industrialisation and scientific dominance: "Where the word filth once suggested, with its moralist air, the evils of the flesh, the word toxic now condemns the chemical evils of the industrial world." Like my patient Angelo, there is what Dr Kerryn Phelps calls "an emerging mainstream" that resort to actions that give them a feeling of personal purity, especially when faced with a world of endless complexity and a vague sense that nature is being corrupted.

What was interesting about my patient Angelo was that he was no inner city hippy and nor did he come from a culture that actively promoted environmentalism or a strong connection with nature and healthy food. He had absorbed it from the prevailing zeitgeist.

I was surprised Angelo kept attending appointments, although I knew his income protection might kick up a fuss if he didn't. After six sessions he agreed to trial a low dose of the gentlest anti-depressant. He acquired a pill cutter from the pharmacist to break the pill into quarters. The amount was bordering on a homeopathic dose but it was better than nothing.

Shifting patient attitudes is often a game of politics, where pressure groups in the form of relatives who hold influence in the lives of patients require mobilisation. Even for the sickest of patients, the status quo can be the safe bet. Partners and children were the most influential, but Angelo was adamant that I wasn't allowed to involve them.

He stopped the tablet within days after he experienced some nausea and a sensation he described as "mental numbness". Antidepressants have their share of side effects but for Angelo many of his complaints were a function of his own attitudes and anxiety about how the tablets might affect his physiology.

"I could feel something foreign inside of me," he said when explaining why he stopped taking the medication. "It was a kind of violence."

I found it difficult not to see Angelo's reaction as melodramatic, but I heard similar things from patients who were fearful of vaccination. They perceived it as a kind of unwanted assault from conspiratorial forces of power, a kind of pharmaceutical/medical industrial complex.

A breakthrough came several months later when his daughter Jessica arrived at an appointment. She was a cheerful young woman completing university studies. Angelo was jittery when Jessica sat in our consultation. I jumped on the opportunity and asked her to outline what she thought Angelo's problems were. Jessica was taken aback, not expecting that I might want her candid opinions. She looked furtively towards her father, hoping for some kind of permission. There was no gesture from Angelo, but Jessica apologised to him first, before launching into an extended account of what she described as her father's symbolic death.

"We are grieving for him really," said Jessica, holding back tears while reaching for the tissue box on my desk. "He is there physically, but not much else. I eat donuts at home sometimes to annoy him, get some kind of reaction."

"Yes, that is a terrible thing Jessica," said Angelo, shaking his head, oblivious of the joke. But he was gripping his chair as Jessica spoke, clearly affected.

I assessed Angelo alone after Jessica had revealed the hopelessness he had rendered in the rest of the household. He knew his difficulties affected his wife and daughters, but had underestimated the extent. Nor had he realised they saw his routines and habits as a function of mental illness and not as a flight towards health. The session offered a potential opening for him to reassess his fears surrounding pharmaceuticals.

I opted down a slightly different path and suggested he take the herbal remedy St John's Wort. A flower long believed to have mild anti-depressant properties, I hoped it might function as a placebo. I wasn't convinced the herb had much in the way of active properties – some studies found it effective, others did not – but considered it the equivalent of an integrative approach much like if I involved the pastor or imam in the treatment of a religious believer. Taking something for his mood would also condition Angelo to take a tablet that had more significant psychoactive properties.

Weeks later he had started having some meals with the rest of the family and even attended church like he had done prior to leaving his business. He said he found it terrifying, facing a large crowd of people, many from the Filipino community. He was overwhelmed when a family friend asked him about his business, but his daughter had the awareness to step in and whisk him away.

I convinced Angelo to make another attempt to trial a gentle anti-depressant and perhaps start seeing a psychologist to help make practical plans to break his preoccupation with a skewed idea of health. I sought Jessica's help to reassure him when he suffered the inevitable side effects and wanted to stop. Two further sessions involved long discussions reassuring Angelo of the ultimate safety of the anti-depressants, especially at such a low dose. His worldview of a malevolent power complex corrupting the purity of the natural world, which included his own biology, was steadily being chipped away. There was no need to break it entirely, just allow it to sit alongside treatment.

My aim was to help Angelo understand that his notion of authenticity was deeply isolating and his true self was utterly connected to those he loved and served. Meaning did not emerge from exclusively looking inward. Angelo remains on the medications for now and has even mentioned returning to part-time financial planning. I myself had long stopped searching for some elusive essence of who I am and have any notion of self reflected back from the affection of my family and gratitude of patients.

# 5

# SECULAR PRIESTS:
# MENTAL HEALTH AS MORALITY

There are many days when I feel like my work is no different from that of a priest. I am not wearing any colourful robes and there is a room with a comfy chair instead of a booth. But I am inundated with patients walking into my room with their relatives and confessing their sins.

"Doctor, I get angry too much and the kids are scared of me," said a father who worked as an office manager.

"I need help with losing too much money on the pokies," said a single mother employed part-time in a pharmacy.

"I am filled with guilt about not being a good wife," said a manifestly depressed middle-aged woman no longer interested in intimacy.

While there is a minority of patients who may have sought some counsel from religious authorities, the vast majority will instinctively head for the soft, non-threatening ambience of the therapist's waiting room.

During a rotation working in one of the oldest psychiatrist

asylums in Australia, Rozelle Hospital, I remember a sign on the wall of the nursing station. It was subtle but unmissable, sticky taped and its message marked in green texta. Personality disorder = dickhead, it said. It is an old joke in mental health, but like stereotypes and effective humour, its power lies in exposing a partial truth.

Personality disorder refers to people whose coping behaviours are dysfunctional enough that they cannot function in relationships or working roles consistently. Under pressure or crisis, we can all exhibit some traits that might fall into such categories, such as being extra sensitive to criticism, feeling abandoned or rejected easily or not having appropriate empathy towards others – a feature of narcissism or anti-social personalities. But those who are considered personality disordered do so consistently over a long period and leave a trail of personal destruction in their wake.

The sign comparing such a person to a dickhead is apt because it neatly captures a dramatic shift in how we view our inner selves. Over the last century we have shifted from having characters to personalities. The term character has moral overtones in that you can be good or bad. During elections for example there is a great focus on the characters of the candidates and to what extent they are morally suitable. Personality has a different connotation. Its overtones have more to do with self-presentation. As a result, much behavior previously considered immoral or wrong now falls under disorder. We seamlessly blend moral problems with questions surrounding mental health.

Of the seven deadly sins, pride and envy effectively equate to narcissism, gluttony is an eating disorder, sloth might be construed as a dependent personality disorder, and acting out in anger might be called an intermittent explosive disorder. I have to confess when I first heard the term for anger outbursts, I assumed it referred to an aggressive diarrhoea.

*The New York Times* columnist David Brooks writes in his bestselling book *The Road to Character* that words like 'sin', 'soul' and 'redemption' are echoes of a distant vernacular but are now diluted. Sin, for example, is more likely to be used in the context of desserts than sex, a pointer that food is increasingly a way people express their value systems. Brooks makes reference to a study by American sociologist Christian Smith, in which he asked college students about moral dilemmas and found they often lacked the language to consider the issues at hand. This raises the question whether in replacing or at least creating a parallel system of mental health to deal with moral questions, whether we even have the words to grapple with morality anymore.

If we use the term 'character', most of us are likely to be referring to a friend or acquaintance who is a bit quirky or offbeat, perhaps the one who shuns the norms of society and lives in a Buddhist temple for six months or has a particular fascination with old shoes. But the historical meaning of character in relation to building intelligent, positive habits instead of destructive ones are what American philosopher John Dewey calls the 'interpenetration of habits'.

My job as a psychiatrist is wholly concerned with determining whether my patients are healthy or sick. To what extent are they impaired or unfit and how might I relieve their psychic suffering as a result? Moral guilt and blame seem at odds with helping or healing. The connotations of morality are as it relates to actions and its effects on other people, whereas good health is oriented to the self. This is often the basis of criticism of the therapeutic paradigm in its elevation of self-fulfilment over obligation to others.

Oxford Professor of philosophy, Michael Martin, argues in a

book called *Morality and Mental Health* that several themes bridge the two topics.

One is that sound morality is healthy. Moral attitudes tend to overlap with mental health. For example, if a murderer is upset, depressed and feeling guilt because of his crime and being placed in jail, this is hardly mental illness but an appropriate reaction to his circumstances. Alternatively feeling on a high after receiving gratitude for good work might appear to an outsider as appearing elevated in mood.

We are also largely responsible for ensuring or bettering our health, both mental and physical. As a result sickness does not automatically excuse wrongdoing.

The final overlapping theme is that moral values permeate definitions of mental illness. For instance, the criteria that determine whether you are depressed or not must include an inability to maintain relationships or purposeful activity such as paid work. The severity exists on a spectrum but this definition implies that a functional human being engages in relationships and works, a definition which is laden with values. It's rooted in Freud's belief that a functional adult was able "to love and to work".

A psychiatrist has enormous power in being able to both define a disorder and then treat it. This power is most profound when a patient is scheduled and treated against their will in public hospitals. It is perhaps not a surprise that psychiatry has abused its power or been co-opted by governments. The abuse has varied from the Soviets creating disorders such as 'delusions of capitalism' to the construction of illnesses in the 19th century such as drapetomania – the desire of slaves to escape from their owner.

For all the promotion of good mental health aimed at reducing the stigma of emotional disorders, it is worth bearing in mind that the line between mental health and social tyranny has historically been small. Given the dominant paradigm of political opposition often overlaps with identity politics, there is a risk of the notion of psychological harm being co-opted to assist in this project.

Sometimes it can be difficult to avoid bringing in my values to consultations, especially for patients whose actions clearly cross moral boundaries. But the malleability of some patient's actions and my profession's powers in altering behaviour biochemically has softened my views around bad behaviour.

A particular patient I treated in a regional town was a case in point. Harry was in his early thirties and worked in a strategic managerial role for a major dairy producer. Broad in shoulders and accent, he was by no means a country bumpkin. He grew up on the land in a pastoralist family. His parents and grandparents ran cattle and sheep. They were wealthy and well connected. He had attended a Sydney boarding school and occasionally expressed envy of the large proportion of his friends making a motza in the big city financial industry, a staple career of the male, private school boys.

When he first came to me, the letter from his general practitioner bordered on cryptic: "Dear Dr Ahmed, Thank you for assessing this patient for some problems he is having in his personal life. He has asked to see you."

I was both intrigued and annoyed. The letter alluded that it hadn't been the family doctor's idea for Harry to see me and also implied that he wanted to use me in counselling Harry for his life's difficulties.

"Doc, this might be a strange one for you," Harry began with a wry grin. He sat diagonally opposite me on an adjustable office chair.

"There are no limits to strange in this job," I quipped.

"Um, how do I say this, I keep cheating on my wife," he said. "I'm not proud of it, but it keeps happening."

I nodded. "Tell me more. I'm interested in how you think I might be able to help," I said.

My initial reaction was that here was a case of somebody not willing to take responsibility for his actions, lacking all insight into the moral nature of his behaviour and hoping to acquire a medical condition through which he could happily deflect any sense of personal blame. And why would he present to a psychiatrist and not a priest or a good friend? He was the sort of person who would traditionally have had a drink with a mate and volunteered his problems over a schooner of beer.

Harry had been married to his schoolteacher wife for seven years and they had two children. He didn't express any particular dissatisfaction with the marriage, but he found himself binge drinking on the weekend, usually in the company of friends, and then being unable to resist sexual opportunities on offer, aided by the town's status as a university centre overflowing with available young women. It didn't help his problems that he had been a high level rugby player in his youth and still had a muscular frame. During the week he was able to perform in his job without much difficulty and his wife was aware of only one extra-marital encounter from several years prior.

"What's made you want help for this now?" I asked him.

His father, who Harry described as supportive but often authoritarian and occasionally verbally abusive had been diagnosed with bowel cancer. His father didn't mind a drink. Harry described his earliest memory of his father sitting at a table describing in detail a prize bottle of brandy. But he was not an alcoholic. The severity of his father's cancer was not yet clear, but it appeared to bring up questions of mortality and, in turn, morality for Harry.

Harry had always had problems with controlling his impulses, often getting in trouble at school and struggling with a gambling habit for several years while at university. He once lost a thousand dollars in one sitting on the poker machines at a Sydney sports club. But he was able to recover and soldier on, ultimately landing on his feet in an important job. I wondered if becoming a father created any conflicts for him.

"No, I love being a dad. I manage the soccer team of the older boy. We have a great relationship. I just don't want to hurt their mother," he said, becoming more emotional as the interview progressed. We were both leaning forward towards each other, a sign of a good therapeutic rapport.

Harry did not have a disorder that might fit neatly into psychiatric classification. I could call it an alcohol misuse disorder, where the alcohol consumption was not regular and didn't disrupt his functioning significantly but did put him into risky, harmful situations. He had some features of a narcissistic personality, where he lacked a degree of empathy and didn't entirely account for the effect of his actions upon loved ones. He had a problem with impulse control, another issue that would traditionally have been associated with character, but one that fell on the margins of psychiatric medicalisation. The primary, formal impulse disorder in psychiatry was considered to be gambling, which Harry did have a history of.

After the first appointment I bluntly told him my skills didn't have much to offer, that his problems were controllable actions and that he could simply take himself out the situations in which he was more likely to misbehave. I didn't call him a dickhead, but it was what I was thinking. In short, he could keep it in his pants.

He was aware that limiting his opportunities was an obvious answer but worried that doing that would drastically dilute his social life with his circle of friends, many of whom did not yet have children. There was an element of Harry's behaviour that fell into the man-child category, but he did turn up seeking help, so I didn't want to be too harsh. I suggested he see a psychologist with a view to recognising his triggers surrounding drinking alcohol given that was the biggest contributor to his adultery.

Several months had passed when he reappeared, informing me that he had been to several sessions with a psychologist and even consulted with a local priest but he felt there was something primitive and uncontrollable in his actions. This seemed fanciful to me. He had improved and had very few extra-marital liaisons, despite having regular opportunities, but he gave a history of being ruled by impulses. I considered a frontal lobe disorder of the brain whereby some kind of injury, usually a head injury from a fall or car accident, causes damage to the part of the brain and alters our personality and, in particular, our impulses. This was unlikely in Harry, especially given he had no such problems at work.

Harry came to me relatively early in my career as a specialist. He was not the type of patient who would ever present to a public hospital. I went against my practice and tried placing him on a low dose of anti-depressant and a mood stabiliser. I knew this combination would likely reduce his impulsivity.

Despite their name, anti-depressants were often better for treating anxiety, reducing frustration tolerance and modifying impulsivity. I genuinely thought the medication might help, but was slightly uncomfortable with what was loosely the treatment of formal psychiatric illness.

I did not see Harry for over a year and was due to stop visiting the regional town. During one of my last practice days, I arrived from the airport and there he was sitting in my waiting room, dressed in a suit and an Akubra Stockman.

"You fixed me, doc. I've been going great guns since you started me on those tablets. I feel so relaxed and can have a couple of drinks without doing anything," Harry said, positively beaming. "I was hoping I could try coming off 'em."

I wasn't surprised that the medications did help, but didn't expect him to remain on them given the potential side effects. I suggested he try and reduce the dose or stop one of the tablets entirely. There was a chance that he had established new patterns of behaviour that may be reflected in modified neurochemistry in the brain, although dramatic change was optimistic. I bid my goodbyes to Harry, wished him well and he presented me with a bottle of French wine as a parting gift. I felt more comfortable that there was nothing wrong or unethical about medically improving aspects of personality that may also fall in the realm of character and morality.

A research group at The Oxford Centre for Neuroethics is investigating this possibility: to what extent can we use pharmaceuticals for moral improvement. Research associate Brian Earp told Quartz magazine: "Imagine a psychopath who doesn't have the ability to deal with other people's pain and, because of that, is more likely than others to commit violent crime. If we could treat psychopaths to make them feel more empathy, then surely that would be worthwhile. The same is true for those who experience blinding rage, and do terrible things in the heat of their anger."

An Australian philosopher from the same department, Julian Savulescu, also argues that we have a moral responsibility to use drugs to promote better performance in many aspects of the human economy. The drug most commonly mentioned in this debate is modafinil, which is a wakefulness drug licensed for use for narcolepsy, which is when people have a condition where they can suddenly fall asleep. Savulescu argues that modafinil could be used safely in a host of endeavours, from employees trading stocks to surgery, and it would be beneficial for humanity as a whole.

His pronouncements should make many of us wary and imagine the emergence of Aldous Huxley's *Brave New World* as a potential and imminent reality; a world where we biochemically enhance the population to become, in Oprah Winfrey speak, our 'best selves', at least in terms of economic and social performance.

The bad news, or perhaps good news depending on where you stand, is that self improvement through medication is already happening. There is a fine line between performance or moral enhancement as opposed to treating psychological illness. As Israeli philosopher, Yuval Harari, writes in his book *Homo Deus: A Brief History of Tomorrow*, 'no clear line exist between healing and upgrading'.

There used to be a view in psychiatry that it was not possible to modify personality disorders, or features of character, but it is impossible to remove aspects of personality from mental health presentations.

For example, if you are a perfectionist, obsessional and perhaps a little avoidant, your internalising traits make you far more likely to become depressed at some stage in your life. The idea promoted by some aspects of mental health advocacy, not to mention the pharmaceutical industry, that people fall under depression much like catching a cold, is fiction, although the notion can be useful to reduce stigma and encourage people to seek help.

I have used modafinil on several occasions for patients who struggle with excessive tiredness or are so wracked with anxiety that they can barely get out of bed. None of these patients has narcolepsy and they can't claim the subsidy for buying the drug, but almost each and every one of them is thankful for beginning the tablet and attribute dramatic improvements in their lives to the medication. They need not be elite workers, although modafinil is used by sections of the military including the marines who assassinated Osama Bin Laden in the dead of night in Pakistan.

The transformation that occurred in these patients was both satisfying and troubling. Their relatives, bosses or teachers often refer to such patients as "a new person", expressed in positive terms. Suddenly they are more social, charismatic, display better business acumen and improved sexual prowess.

There was something almost suspicious about such a level of improvement that challenged notions of the continuity of the self. It also implied a level of biological determinism given that our vulnerabilities from our development clearly leave a biological signature seemingly modified through chemical alteration. The groundbreaking book written over twenty years ago by Brown University Professor Peter Kramer, Listening to Prozac, captures this anxiety felt by prescribers.

> I was suspicious of Prozac, as if I had just taken on a co-therapist whose charismatic style left me wondering whether her magic was wholly trustworthy... It is all very well for a drug to do small things: to induce sleep, to allay anxiety, to ameliorate a well recognised syndrome. But for a drug's effect to be so global- to extend to social popularity, business acumen, self-image, energy, flexibility, sexual appeal- touches too closely about medication for the mind.

Professor Kramer also coined the term "better than well" in reference to the fine line between improving the symptoms of illness and enhancing the social, academic or occupational performance of an otherwise healthy person.

Anti-depressants are the most widely used drugs in mental health. Australia has the second highest usage in the developed world with only Iceland popping happy pills more enthusiastically. The use has doubled between the years 2001 and 2011, to the point where eighty nine people out of a thousand were prescribed the class of medications. But as Kramer's analysis illustrates, there can be a fine line between treating illness and enhancing performance. Their use can arouse heated passions given the overlap with modifying aspects of the self. This is even a bigger challenge for drugs like Ritalin, dexamphetamine or modafinil, which can improve focus, concentration or alertness for otherwise functional people. They are also accessible online. It is a debate and potential cultural transformation that we are in the early stages of. The most obvious area where my work overlaps with character and morality are dealings with the law. One patient I treated was a young computer professional prone to taking his clothes off inappropriately, something that provoked disgust and called his character into question.

Archie was a computer programmer in his early twenties referred by his defence lawyer. It was my job to assess him over the course of two hours and give an opinion as to what extent his actions were related to a mental illness and whether any condition was modifiable through appropriate treatment. Medical training didn't entirely prepare me for the game of the law, a place where legal truths didn't always correspond to medical or scientific ones. Finding a balance between advocating as strongly as possible for the person in front of me sometimes felt in conflict with a doctor's obligations to the court and to society. Archie's future depended upon the contents of my report.

Archie had immaculately trimmed sideburns that he grew right to his jawline, implying a degree of obsessionality and perfectionism.

He was clearly anxious – he was trembling as he sat down. I could see beads of sweat on his forehead and he avoided eye contact.

I read the police facts sheet, which outlined him running around naked in a shopping centre car park and scaring a middle-aged woman carrying her groceries before being discovered by security guards. He was taken to the police station thereafter for questioning.

I looked over at him as he sat opposite me with his head bowed, a picture of humiliation and embarrassment.

According to the police sheet, he had also been charged and fined for being naked in public only weeks earlier, on New Year's Eve. Suspecting he may suffer from a sexual disorder, I asked him to tell me about this earlier episode first.

"I'm really just an IT guy, not some weird sex freak. I can't explain what happened," he protested, shaking his head. I knew from experience that being an IT guy and weird sex freak were not mutually exclusive, but I told him I just wanted to hear, in his words, what happened that night.

"Well," he said hesitantly, "I guess I was still trying to get over Samira."

"Samira?"

"My girlfriend. Ex-girlfriend," he corrected himself.

I nodded and left an encouraging space for him to fill.

"We broke up last September."

"Uh-huh."

"She didn't think we had a future. Her family are Lebanese Christians, and I'm…" He gestured at his skin and trailed off.

"Not Maronite Christian, I'm guessing," I said, managing to

extract a wry smile from Archie. "So, how did you meet?"

"We work together. She sits in the cubicle next to me."

"Still?" I asked, as neutrally as possible. "That must be hard."

Archie nodded while frowning, and told me about getting uncharacteristically drunk on several occasions at Friday night work drinks, in the hope that Samira might feel sympathy and give him much desired attention. It didn't happen and Archie felt rejected once more, often struggling to complete tasks with his usual efficiency. His colleagues became worried and advised him to minimise the time he spent speaking to her. His immediate manager even suggested he take a week off and perhaps go on holiday, but Archie felt it was an over-reaction.

I wondered whether he had a streak of self-flagellation – a desire to humiliate himself that perhaps played out in his incidents of public nudity. After all, he didn't seem to get much pleasure from them.

Shortly before the New Year's incident he had started learning to use the dating application Tinder, hoping he would summon the courage to meet someone. He showed me the photo he used, his favourite digital photo, the one where he only had a partial smile and his sideburns were thick and bushy. He wanted to attract smart girls who might be interested in technology, although he qualified this by saying the technology side wasn't essential.

"I wasn't wanting sex or anything," he continued, bowing his head. "But I didn't really want to be at home with my father either."

He signalled there might be some tension with his father. I was conscious that as an authority figure with some power over his life, there was a risk Archie might see and react to me a little like his father. He explained that his mother and older brother, Ashok, had undertaken a brief trip to Hyderabad for a relative's wedding, leaving Archie alone in the house with his father.

Archie said he set his search criteria on Tinder to girls in their twenties within ten kilometres of his location, and within hours met one. I nodded vigorously in an attempt to hide my wonder at the brave, new technological world of dating, despite being only a decade or so older than Archie.

"How did it go?" I asked.

Archie became more guarded and spoke more softly. He said they drank several glasses of bourbon and cola at the middle bar, the one overlooking the water skiers in the local river, before driving to a car park adjacent to the water. Archie was anxious that he was still a virgin and did not want to reveal it to his casual love interest. I thought it was unusual in this day and age that his relationship with Samira was not consummated and wondered whether it was due to her religious beliefs.

Archie at no stage referred to the girl by name. He said they kissed for a little while, but he couldn't stop thinking about Samira. So he drove his Tinder girlfriend home. All he could think about was Samira. He wondered who she was with, whether she might have met someone new and the likelihood that she wasn't thinking about Archie at all. He felt gutted, demoralised and overwhelmed with grief.

He remembered parking the car in a laneway and playing some music. He couldn't remember the song. His next memory was being outside the car naked and hearing the shouts and laughter of men in a passing car, with the flash of phone cameras attempting to photograph his humiliation and digitally share it for time immemorial.

"They were trying to take photos on their phones. They said they'd put it on Facebook," said Archie. "I jumped back into my car and put my clothes on."

This is where the police facts sheet began recording events and history, stating that Archie was seen at around 2.30am in a narrow lane standing naked by his car and carrying his clothes in his hands. The driver's door was ajar. He was alone, and there was no reference to him masturbating, which was important in formulating the diagnosis.

"Do you have any memory of being aroused during this period?" I interrupted, attempting to establish whether sexual deviance was a factor.

"No way, I was really upset." Archie was emphatic, making clearer eye contact.

Treating and assessing patients with sexual deviance disorders was particularly confronting. I remembered visiting a paedophile unit at Long Bay jail during my training as a psychiatrist. My wife was pregnant with our first child, which we had just learned was a little girl. I had never been so repulsed by a patient as I was when interviewed a gaunt, wrinkled man in his fifties who had worked as a clerk at the Roads and Traffic Authority throughout his life prior to his arrest. Maintaining empathy was a challenge. I felt more compassion for the murderers I had treated. I hoped Archie was nothing like that.

Exhibitionism, better known as flashing – becoming sexually excited while exposing one's genitals to unsuspecting strangers, usually children or women – may not seem very serious. As a high school student walking through Sydney's Hyde Park, I was familiar with dishevelled men in overcoats suddenly showing off their wares to passing students. But I knew any legal opposing counsel would closely scrutinise the possibility of exhibitionism because it is difficult to treat, and has the same high rates of recidivism as paedophilia. In its worst forms, the intrusiveness combined with the sexual nature overlapped with assault. Archie's episodes would be no laughing matter in court.

One of the key questions in Archie's case was whether the strangers stumbled upon him or the other way around. The police statement implied the strangers were shocked and amused by Archie's antics to the point where they attempted to take photos on their phone. There was no evidence that Archie went looking for them, or that he experienced any pleasure.

I asked him about internet pornography consumption and he said it was occasional, perhaps once or twice a month, which was well below the average of twice a week for men. His habit was prudish by comparison. But if his behaviour wasn't driven by sexual deviance, what was it?

Archie was born in a Bangalore hospital as the second son of an accountant father and mother who worked as a teacher. Before it became the Silicon Valley of the developing world, the city was an industrial hub and his father worked for an automotive parts company in its auditing division.

The family migrated when Archie was six. I identified with him attending a western Sydney school at that age, its mix of newly arrived immigrants and working class whites. He didn't describe it as being difficult but said he kept to himself, often sitting alone in the playground. He developed more friends in high school through an interest in sport and technology. It was the dawn of Google and Facebook just as he entered his final years of high school and an interest in computers was not as socially stigmatised.

Archie remembered little of his early childhood, but said his relatives always commented on him being much quieter than his older brother. He said his first memory was of his brother spilling a drink on him while they sat and watched television. He said he cried, but what he really remembered was his father getting angry with his mother about it and shouting at her.

I asked him whether his father was often that angry.

"Yes, unfortunately, it was his way," he said, his voice and tone becoming more brittle.

Archie said that his father was occasionally violent towards his mother and also to the boys, usually slapping or pushing them. He was also a keen drinker of Scotch whisky, which I knew to be the alcoholic poison of choice for the Indian middle classes. He didn't describe anybody in the family having any serious injuries from such incidents, but described a menacing, unforgiving environment in the household.

"I never really felt comfortable," he said, tears welling in his eyes. "I just got used to it, I think."

Archie could not remember if he had any panic attacks as a teenager and denied any thoughts of self-harm, but he vividly described coming home late in the afternoons and rushing to his room during his youth. He tried to avoid any confrontation or meetings with his father, who he experienced as a conservative disciplinarian. He described frantically, almost violently, taking his clothes off and sitting on his bed wearing only shorts, a tracksuit bottom or even just his underpants. He said it relieved his tension. He hadn't done anything like that for many years, not since he had begun university.

A phone conversation with Archie's older brother, Ashok, after the interview underlined that Archie had always been a shy, reserved boy who, in spite of a social awkwardness was ultimately able to make a small circle of friends. Ashok related his own story of discovering Archie sitting on his bed dressed only in his underpants once while his parents were arguing loudly. Ashok came to check on his younger brother, but closed the door thinking that Archie may have been masturbating.

While he confirmed their parents often fought, he was eager to impress that it was not violent or threatening. Their father was the traditional, Asian male coming to terms with living in a more permissive culture where his occupational status was much diminished after migration. Ashok also related that he himself was about to marry, which I suspected was significant and may have heightened Archie's sense of loss over his relationship breakdown.

I thought the description of his behaviour as a child was an unusual coping mechanism whereby patients virtually lost consciousness, although technically the way they processed sensory data was disrupted. The sensory disturbance was usually a way of coping with serious trauma, particularly rape or sexual abuse. The behaviour repeated itself sometimes in other situations of adversity. The brain switches into the mode as a way of coping with stressful events, often to the person's detriment.

In its most extreme form, patients could appear like entirely different people. The technical term for the notion of multiple personality disorder was "dissociative identity disorder". There was no suggestion Archie suffered from having multiple personalities, but he gave a convincing past history of having dissociated.

I felt I had enough information to at least tell a convincing story that Archie was not a future risk and could be managed with greater psychological input and perhaps a low dose medication to reduce anxiety. Few magistrates wanted to put away first offenders, particularly if presented with a viable, alternative proposal.

Days later, accompanied by his parents and older brother, Archie stood in front of the magistrate in Parramatta District Court. His mother was dressed in a beige, silk sari and held back her tears. The hearing was brief, which came as a relief to all. I was not required to give testimony and had avoided being ticked off by an opposing barrister, which was the case in a handful of previous court encounters.

"I'm satisfied that according to Dr Ahmed's report that you have an anxiety disorder. I suggest you find better ways to deal with it than exposing yourself in public, young man. Good day to you. Next," said the wigged judge, before ceremonially banging his hammer.

I felt a surge of joy for Archie, confirmation that I had perhaps identified with him a little too much. His South Asian heritage, surly father and western Sydney upbringing mirrored my own experience.

Archie had probably begun to dissociate as a teenager as a way of coping with his parents' conflict at home. There was a good chance he was in a spontaneous trance when he rushed to his room and flung off his clothes. Having always been shy and withdrawn, he could not find outlets of communicating his distress, which lay at the heart of a healthy psyche. When he was faced with an altogether different trauma in adulthood, that of his first, broken, romantic relationship, he returned unconsciously to prior ways of coping. Melodramatic songs in the car seemed to be a major trigger. This linked the car park to the laneway during New Year's Eve, which were both echoes of his teenage years when as a quiet, scared child he tore his clothes off after school as his silent protest towards his parents' imminent conflict.

Archie's case was an example of what could easily be seen as a moral or question of character falling under the lens of mental illness. His actions elicited disgust but his deviant behaviour was highly treatable and he has functioned well afterwards, having visited a psychologist for several sessions and ceasing a low dose anti-depressant after six months. His case is relatively novel, but the most common cases are of socially disadvantaged boys with troubled upbringings who are impulsive and use drugs to varying degrees. Usually under the influence of substances, they act out through assault or low-grade robberies. The majority of them can be helped with low dose medications, much like Harry's impulsive adultery was fixed.

I offer a detailed treatment plan which magistrates usually agree to. I agree to inform the Court if the defendant does not abide by the suggested plan. In such an arrangement, the magistrate is playing his part in administering mental health treatment and psychological experts help uphold law and order. Underlying the process was a sophisticated view of human nature that combined a moral, religious view of man with psychological science. Archie had a moral duty to improve his coping behaviours.

Be it Archie or Harry, the medications did have the power to modify behaviour but the improvements rarely continued unless the patient was able to learn better coping skills, usually in the form of improved communication, which didn't always have to be verbal. For this reason I was sceptical of Harry's ability to remain well given he was so reliant on the medications alone. The author Karen Blixen said, "All sorrows can be borne if you put them into a story or tell a story about them." But when people don't have the tools to tell their story, the story tells them via the plethora of symptoms that fall under the lens of mental illness.

My role as an amalgam of priest and medical practitioner was to intervene and help patients articulate their story. This went beyond confession alone and sometimes involved powerful medications, the effects of which lay on the margins of improving illness but also enhancing performance and character.

# 6

# ANGRY WHITE MEN

In descriptions of his early life studying in the United Kingdom, celebrated author Salman Rushdie recounts how his image of Britain was shaped through the writing of great novelists and philosophers, from Shakespeare to James Joyce to Keats. He imagines a sophisticated, high-minded society where the ordinary populace makes literary references and debates democratic principles. His view was cemented as a youth by the dominance of colonial institutions in India.

You can imagine his surprise when his first sighting of the English in their natural environment was an intoxicated man in a football jersey vomiting in a street alley.

My mother had a similar experience. The eldest of eight children, she was raised in a village but educated in a secondary boarding school and city university. She worked as an English teacher at a prestigious primary school before my parents migrated to Australia. While a great deal of their education depended upon rote learning, she had nevertheless absorbed a considerable appreciation of English literature. My mother took great pride in being able to recite her favourite quote from Macbeth: "Tomorrow and tomorrow and tomorrow, Creeps in this petty pace from day to day. To the last syllable of recorded time. And all our yesterdays are like lighted fools. The way to dusty death."

Pregnant with my younger sister and due to begin a very different life in an unknown land, she brushed up on her English literature hoping it may be of use after arrival in Sydney. She hoped she might casually throw in a sonnet from *A Midsummer Night's Dream* to make the trip through customs smoother or use a verse from one of Coleridge's poems during her first job interview. Alas, the opportunity never eventuated. Instead she experienced an onslaught of Australian larrikin, working-class culture in all its glory, both warm and coarse.

"What's that dot on your head, love?" she was asked innocently by the man who presented her with a Medicare card.

"Your kid is a bit of a slow coach," our first babysitter, Doreen, casually instructed my mother in relaying my journey to school.

Such blunt, abrupt interaction, seemingly free of boundaries and Shakespearean prose was a challenge for my mother. It left her in a degree of fear of venturing outside lest a new, curious creature of western Sydney would accost her and ask uncomfortable questions.

I encountered an awe and curiosity of Western culture during family visits to Bangladesh every few years. I remember as a young adult meeting a fresh-faced boy, part way through university, who asked me questions about Jane Austen and what I thought about *Pride and Prejudice*. This was someone who had barely ventured out of a Bangladeshi village. I explained to him that nobody actually read those books voluntarily, but only because they were compulsory texts for high school examinations. I also admitted that I didn't even do that and just memorised the cheat notes. He shook his head in disappointment before walking away despondently.

Such interactions showed me the reverence many people from developing countries held for Western culture, even if it was based on Hollywood or consumer culture. The admiration was held in combination with resentment, especially for what was perceived as the historical injustice of colonialism. But the appreciation of culture through great literature was a marker of a broader acknowledgement of the achievements surrounding democracy, the rule of law and a free press.

The same boy who asked me about Jane Austen was also a great devotee of debating. He joked that few people in Bangladesh could engage in reasoned debate that didn't descend into personal attacks or violent reprisal. I was embarrassed and shown up for taking a great deal of my political and social environment for granted, yet the boy had never been overseas.

This admiration and elevated expectations on the part of some new migrants was partially tainted by initial interactions before new migrants understood Australian norms. Thereafter they better recognised that what first appeared as rude or racist was often a display of a unique Australian warmth and different attitudes surrounding hierarchy and authority. Initial interactions new migrants had were inevitably with those of the white working class and, to this day, the interplay between newly arrived migrants and the working classes form the political fault lines of the day, from attitudes to refugees to views around population. These first impressions ran true with Mark Twain's observation that Australia was an entire nation of the working class.

Growing up in the disadvantaged suburb of Toongabbie in western Sydney, my upbringing combined an uptake of some aspects of Australian battler culture with a mild disdain and outright reverse racism for other traits such as the limited cuisine, poor fashion sense and devotion to gambling.

I had the attitude that the houses of white people smelt like dog, which was what my parents also believed. The opinion incorporated the prejudice that white Australians were more interested in their pets than their extended families. Ethnic groups were idealised in terms of their devotion to tight, extended families and the associated support and obligation that came with them. The 1980s, which was when we arrived in Sydney, were still early in the rapid devastation that the working class family experienced, arguably through the social laissez faire movements of the immediate decades prior in combination with the welfare state.

But regular stories of divorce, single parents and teenage pregnancies cemented this association of social disintegration with whites. The prejudice I absorbed from my family and Bangladeshi community, in its worst form, associated poor white people as having uncouth, animal natures.

I inherited a love of rugby league from friends in primary school. I engaged in the ritual verbal abuse of the referee during some weekend games I attended with my father. I enjoyed and felt proud of his passion that bordered on maniacal rage. Our love of footy was one aspect of the culture that we were fully integrated into. Most other aspects such as gambling, alcohol, the local RSL club, and meat and two veg cuisine remained out of bounds. We almost never ate out, gambling and alcohol were against our religion, and virtually every home-cooked meal was curry and rice.

My sudden elevation to an elite private school during high school exposed me to a greater slice of social class in Australia. Initially intimidating, performing well academically and athletically was a rapid way of being accepted and celebrated. I felt more convinced of the country's egalitarian, socially mobile spirit. The so-called rich and powerful didn't seem particularly different. Instead of getting drunk with beer, they did it with wine. They had more refined table manners and supported a rugby union team instead of league. There was no appropriate accent required, but a better pronunciation of vowels helped. The barriers to entry to Australia's establishment were hardly insurmountable. You just needed a bit of money, know the right utensils to use and make some occasional references to good wine.

There were still few people with the cultural sophistication my mother had hoped for as a staple of Western life, but I found this attractive given I could not access the high culture of my Bengali ancestry either. I could barely speak the language. My inevitable philistinism was no barrier to local social climbing. It was in fact an aid. Australia was less about social class and more about the American notion of status, which was a matter of self-presentation and more crucially related to what people think of you.

But I also experienced a degree of disdain for people living in the outer suburbs in high school that increased my sympathies for my locality. On the way to the school's annual rowing regatta the other students would cheer my name when the bus passed a sign to Toongabbie. Few of my classmates had any knowledge of the western suburbs or the people inhabiting them, an early lesson in the segregation the sprawling suburbs of Sydney resulted in.

People who lived in Toongabbie were westies, bogans or white trash. To be fair, it was what I thought many of them were too, but hearing it from people who weren't actually living there made me feel guilty for thinking it. Some of my high school friends would joke that every second house in my suburb was burnt down, like the Bronx or south central Los Angeles. I remember protesting and becoming angry, only to watch ambulances and fire engines turn up a few weeks later to a house on our street that did burn down from arson.

But so what? The westies were my neighbours, friends and parents of my former schoolmates. I rode bikes with them to the creek or visited the local shopping centre and loitered in branded tracksuits and sneakers. They were my white trash. I maintained an odd mix of disdain inherited from my ethnic prejudices and newly acquired class sneering with sympathy infused with nostalgia from my childhood adventures. I started seeing them as battlers, contending for the heart of the country against elites wanting to dilute their presence in contemporary Australian life.

I brought this complicated mix of attitudes with me when I consulted white patients from the working class-tradesman, factory workers, truck drivers, secretaries and the unemployed. Much like patients from ethnic groups, they were less likely to present and, if they did, were usually dragged kicking and screaming by a relative or partner.

Unlike wealthier groups, particularly females, who may seek out therapy as part of a project of self-improvement or reinvention, mental health care was often enforced on the poor, whether from work, welfare agencies or the criminal justice system. I was more likely to diagnose men with a mental health condition after seeing them through the courts – the externalisation of distress through aggression or violence is a staple of males.

Just as my ethnic patients were struggling to come to terms with the disintegration of clan and tradition after migration, the working class was losing the scaffolding that gave their lives certainty in the time of my childhood.

Darryl was a difficult patient I had been treating for several years who illustrated the contemporary challenges of his ilk. A stocky man in his forties, he shuffled into each appointment with a walking stick. At first sight, the stick gave him a distinguished quality but then a trace of his bare belly beneath a T-shirt that never quite fit over his bulging gut became visible.

Every appointment would begin the same way.

"How are you travelling, Darryl?" I'd ask.

"Yeah, alright," he'd mumble. "Fucken insurance pissing me off as usual."

Darryl was being funded through worker's compensation after suffering a crush injury to his lower back while lifting crates in a factory. He underwent several operations of inserting plates to metal rods in his spine, to the point where scans of his spine resembled a construction site, but his pain and mobility showed few signs of improvement.

His employer kept him on performing light duties, which was essentially a euphemism for doing the most basic paperwork, but the factory shut down after the manufacturing shifted overseas. He was made redundant but continued to receive compensation payments while he looked for alternative work.

There is an important term in mental health therapy called transference, which refers to the reactions patients arouse in therapists. A good therapist is acutely aware and can counter and override such emotions but also consider them as information about how the patient might affect other people in his life.

My mix of mild disdain and sympathy was awoken each time Darryl visited. He was the epitome of the bogan, the kind of figure the middle classes were desperate not to be associated with, or have their own aspirations for Australian identity tarnished by.

Darryl often wore striped football shirts and a beanie to appointments, even during the height of summer. He said it was to cover an emerging bald spot. He was the only patient to give me a beer coaster as a Christmas present, which I treasure. He even had a name for his penis, which he not so imaginatively called Rod, a name that emerged in our sessions if sexual side effects were being discussed. It was one area of his life where he retained a sense of humour. His childhood memories involved his father taking him to the greyhound races. Darryl was able to give a vivid account of the trips, despite having few words for his emotions.

"The bookies were loud. They'd be screaming the odds before the bloody hare came out. I remember some dog called Leah Turd that won at odds of twenty to one. We won a motza and my dad bought me a massive tub of ice cream," he said with a stealthy grin.

But Darryl's father also suffered a work injury as a carpenter and turned to alcohol. He grew more violent and unable to suppress his rage, started beating his wife, Darryl's mother, a resourceful woman who worked as an aged care nurse and eventually left her husband. Darryl and his younger sister lived with their mother.

Darryl had at least one good decade, when he was married with his first wife, had two young children and a traineeship leading to work with Telecom. He was proud of his time working with the company during the Sydney Olympics, but was made redundant soon after. The marriage ended and his children became more distant. He claimed he could never tell them that it was their mother who was unfaithful, instead unable to temper his anger through vengeful outbursts in the home. His mood only worsened when his factory job was also stymied, first through injury and then through outsourcing.

Now, in my rooms, he was a ball of suppressed rage, usually projected internally in the form of vague thoughts of harming himself, and made worse after he had consumed his evening round of five or six stubbies of beer. He once took an overdose of a prescribed tranquiliser after his new partner threatened to leave him, a prospect that was looking more imminent if he didn't show some improvement.

"It helps me sleep," he says, in reference to his drinking. "If I take more of those pain meds, I can't shit no more."

But despite his efforts to minimise his rage, it would surface at a range of inopportune times. He had been banned from his stepdaughter's primary school for fighting with the teachers, once because he thought too many merit certificates were being handed out – "It makes the kids soft"– and another occasion for verbally abusing the middle-aged woman helping at the pedestrian crossing. "She should have let me cross," he insisted. "There weren't any fucken' cars."

When he drove, Darryl would regularly find himself in heated bouts of road rage, once limping out of his car to threaten another driver for tailing him too closely. He admitted to casually swerving in the direction of people he didn't like the look of.

"I like to give 'em a scare, especially if they look a bit up themself."

On the rare occasions he visited the local shops, he was livid at the demographic changes in the area, a place his extended family had resided in for several generations. So many black and Asian faces, too many fancy designer labels and too few people or organisations backing people like him.

"There's outfits helping out refugees everywhere, on every bloody corner," he railed. "They get extra money at school and everything."

His sense of displacement was most tangibly felt through his regular tussles with the insurance company paying his benefits, attempting to have treatments approved and receive his regular allowance. His mental state was one of free-floating anger that latched to just about any aspect of his immediate environment and identified it as an enemy.

It is difficult not to see the fragmented rage of people like Darryl as being a fundamental factor in the rise of demigods such as Donald Trump, shock developments such as Brexit in Europe or the success and longevity of politicians like Pauline Hanson in Australia. They are the mirror image, the Newtonian reaction to the diffuse resentment of Islamic terrorism, full of dissatisfaction with the "system", but without workable plans. They represent a pining for simpler, collective identities such as nationalism.

Despite the Left building its foundations on the valorisation of the working class throughout the twentieth century, it has now abandoned them to some degree, leaving them free to hold some of the most conservative social views of any group, particularly around race.

Debates around racism are an area where the nose-turning sneering at the working classes is most palpable. The representations of people attending patriotic protests are an obvious example. The protesters are depicted in tattooed, pierced splendour holding angry signs at racist rallies. An accusation of racism is often veiled class sneering using Muslims and other ethnic groups as cover, evidence of French philosopher Pascal Druckner's observation that multiculturalism was sometimes the racism of the anti-racists.

What progressive groups sometimes fail to realise is that by their outward expressions of concern for ethnic groups, and thereby separating themselves from the crass and unsophisticated people who don't express adequate sympathy, progressives are effectively clearing a space for themselves to enjoy the advantages of white privilege.

Patients like Darryl, while an isolated case study, illustrate that no collective group or organisation, other than perhaps the football leagues, is actively representing the white working class. Race-based politics have helped entrench the resentment, for it has given the working class permission to view themselves as an aggrieved, racial group left out in the cold.

Men like Darryl may present to me because they are also the group least likely to manage the gender transition that is necessary for all men in response to changing sexual norms. There is a much greater expectation for all men to be available emotionally to their partners and children not to mention undertake more housework.

Yet most feminist groups and even the psychiatric classification system don't easily incorporate rage as a legitimate expression of emotional distress because there is a belief that it will diminish accountability, particularly in areas such a domestic violence. But as psychiatric patients presenting before the law demonstrate, a more nuanced view that incorporates both responsibility and therapy is possible.

As someone from a very different ethnic background to patients like Darryl, examining racial resentments is of particular interest. Those who express anti-immigration views will often express admiration and affection for authority figures of ethnicity in their lives, such as their family doctor for example, but simultaneously harbour anger to migrants in general.

After the shock of the Brexit outcome in Britain there was a swathe of studies attempting to make links to a wider worldview that supporters may have held, all in a desperate clamour to understand the seemingly inexplicable. A common overlap for supporters was broader authoritarian views, notably predicted by support for the death penalty.

As a psychiatrist, such a turn towards authoritarian certainty makes me think of the place of fathers in my patients' lives. I find it instructive that the handful of my patients with strong ties to anti-immigration groups inevitably had limited or ambivalent links with their father. Darryl did not have any organised links with racist groups but held similar views.

But another patient of mine, Drago, developed strong links to a group similar to Reclaim Australia, wanting to end Muslim immigration. He was a tall, lanky man raised by a devoted single mother. He pined for his Serbian father who lived interstate with a new partner. Drago was referred to me from a disability employment agency because he couldn't hold down a job due to his problems tolerating any kind of frustration. His frustration automatically spilled over into rage rendering him incapable of handling interactions with authority and negotiating with co-workers, a requirement of any workplace. His employment kept getting terminated.

When I asked Drago about hobbies and interests, I discovered he had formed a group with some local friends which they coined the "Slavic brotherhood". His friends and the other members of the group were all raised with little or no presence of a biological father. Did they not notice this overlap, I asked? Drago shrugged and agreed it was something that brought them together, but didn't think it was a big deal.

It is difficult not to see the rise of anti-elite, strongman political figures like Trump as a symbolic yearning for a generation of men derived from the highest proportion of fatherless households in modern history. Without a clear acknowledgement of this deficit or an appropriate channelling into alternative forms of collective identity, such groups will actively look to assert their group identity through outlets of resentment and authoritarian certainty such as anti-immigration organisations or men's rights movements.

Conservative thinker Reihan Salam, author of a book titled *Grand New Party: How Republicans can Win the Working Class and Save*

*The American Dream* writes of an "asymmetrical multiculturalism" whereby minorities are actively encouraged to celebrate their identity and defend their interests while the majority are discouraged from doing it. Outward displays of Italian, Indian or Muslim pride are fine, but if the same occurs for Anglo-Saxons it's regarded as a definite no-no. When whites with many generations of ties wave the national flag or sing the anthem too spiritedly, the fear is that it de-legitimises or dilutes the Australian-ness of other groups.

Salam believes that due to the white majority being denied the option of celebrating their ethnic heritage, they're reduced to championing ideological causes like free speech and the rule of law, stripped of any cultural content. These are notably worthy goals, but as debates around the Racial Discrimination Act in Australia illustrate, they are also indicative of a suppressed nationalism without alternative outlets.

In his book *Angry White Men*, American sociologist Michael Kimmel coins the term "aggrieved entitlement" as a way of describing the losses felt by the white working class, particularly around their power as males in the household, the dilution of their political power in the face of demographic shifts towards ethnic groups and their economic disempowerment in the face of globalisation. He visits characters such as neo-Nazis, wife beaters and angry divorcees to make his point. Kimmel argues such men are failing to make the adjustment to a world where they must be equals instead of the stars of history's arc where they were placed upon a pedestal.

There is certainly truth to this analysis, but it is also in danger of applying one of the most common accusations leftists make of conservatives: that they lack empathy for disadvantaged groups. By continuing to view working or underclass men through the lens of gender or race and not through class or economic entity, it seems that resentments will only be further inflamed and the whittling away of the foundations of the historical Left will continue unabated.

Scottish novelist Andrew O'Hagan in a 2009 George Orwell lecture argued that the English working class is dead, its traditions and values replaced by sentimentality and the illusory promise of credit cards and celebrity. Unlike the Scots and the Irish, who were an innate community held together by songs and speeches about themselves, said O'Hagan, "the English were something else: a riot of individualism, with no sense of common purpose or collective volition as a tribe".

It is possible that Australians exist somewhere in between, with some overlaps with the Scots and Irish in developing a tribal, lighthearted oppositional identity to the English motherland but also exhibiting a greater individualism borne from a stronger cultural influence from America. But with the decline of unions and manufacturing across the Western world, it is difficult to see what traditions, habits and speech bind this amorphous group.

As economic entities the white working class have much in common with newly arrived immigrants, but it is rare that they have the same drive and desperation to rise up the social ladder. The working class is perhaps now a holding bay for those transitioning to the middle class, with a portion falling through the cracks to take their place in the entrenched, welfare-dependent underclass.

An under-recognised aspect of social class and Australian life is noticeable in my work in rural areas. For me this kind of work has been fly-in and fly-out, like so many miners, but wearing cardigans and sweaters instead of fluorescent vests. Working in regional towns is amongst the most rewarding work a doctor can engage in.

There is a uniquely Australian quality to the specialist flying in from the city to a small regional town before flying out on a DASH 8 Qantas flight in the evening. The airline attendants sometimes delayed the flight as they waited for me to rush to the tarmac after finishing my final consultation of the day. Likewise, the rural farmer striving for self-sufficiency against the elements is a quintessential symbol of the modern male and his psychological battles.

The patients are grateful in gaining access to a big city specialist and often the small interventions can transform lives, from beginning a tablet with more tolerable side effects to explaining the origin of their psychic distress. There can be a slapdash element to it given the enormous demand, time constraints and diminished resources. For all its benefits, the service is another example of long-term mental health therapy and its slower unravelling of self-knowledge not being as accessible to the relatively poor.

While many residents in regional towns have lived there for generations, a great deal of the migration is evidence of other trends, from a geographic trickle outwards of the disadvantaged – the disability pension goes a lot further in Bourke than Blacktown – to the white flight from the big cities. When my parents upgraded our family home from Toongabbie to the more leafy suburb of Epping in the early 1990s, I didn't consider that the elderly couple who then moved to the Central Coast was the beginning of a longer term demographic trend.

Many of the patients I see in regional areas are searching. They are sometimes escaping disastrous marriages or family breakdowns, looking to start afresh, perhaps with some extended family support. But a considerable minority are looking for some idea of community that they felt was no longer available in the big city. The idealised image of the tightly knit rural town is no longer what it was. Fewer people make a living from the land, more women have jobs outside the home and people increasingly gain a sense of community from their networks based on mutual interests online. But a common thread that reminded me of the grievances of patients like Darryl was the pining for a sense of the local, a feeling of ownership of their immediate geography.

When supporters of Brexit in England were interviewed, along with views tending to the authoritarian, a common theme was they no longer felt they belonged in the communities they lived in. There were tinges of racism in these stories, with tales of walking to the shops and only hearing Polish or Romanian and no longer recognising others on the street or of shopkeepers calling them by their first name. There is a nostalgia for the past in such stories that borders on delusional, but they are nevertheless the lived experience of many.

Interviews with Londoners who supported Brexit conducted by the BBC illustrated how people celebrated the difference and enjoyed the vitality diversity and migration brought. And the same interviews showed these people were happy to co-exist in separate communities rather than pine for some kind of greater intermingling reminiscent of the past.

Patients like Darryl expressed similar views to the Brexit supporters. Darryl walked to the local shopping centre and became incensed that he felt like a member of a minority group in the place where he had lived for generations. He noticed signs and organisations advocating for newly arrived immigrant groups such as asylum seekers. Any sense of being part of a collective was limited to buying his Lotto ticket or watching his footy team on the weekend. Given Darryl's considerable psychological frailties, he was not indicative of the majority. Most people are adapting, but his inner concerns were pointers to wider trends in dissatisfaction among his demographic group.

British sociologist Will Davies writes that the Brexit campaign slogan "Take Back Control" was ingenious at both a psychological and political level exactly because of the way people like Darryl felt. Their inner experience was one of what is known in psychology as "learned helplessness", where you felt like you were a rickety boat being thrown around in choppy waters. This diagnosis has traditionally been applied to survivors of trauma, particularly women subjected to long-term domestic violence. But in politics as used by Trump, the UK Leave campaign and to some extent Pauline Hanson, the slogan spoke directly to the feeling of inadequacy and embarrassment felt by the white, working class man, and magnified by the class sneering endemic among the inner-city bourgeois. As Davies writes, what such voters crave more than anything else is "the dignity of being self-sufficient, not necessarily in a neo-liberal sense, but certainly in a communal, familial and fraternal sense".

I used to have a view that attempting to engage with patients like Drago and Darryl with a strong psychological angle, attempting to help them gain insight into their coping deficits was doomed to failure, that they were not psychologically minded. But experience has taught me otherwise, that men of limited education, few words and diminished resources were in fact capable of engaging in individual analysis. This did not replace the wider dimension of their position. As American poet Adrienne Rich wrote, "the moment when a feeling enters the body is political". Changes in political economy had affected the working man disproportionately, but the wider project of helping them gain a greater mastery of their emotions and, in turn, their lives, was a worthy social goal. They were reminiscent of the individual versus society being a more relevant struggle for most than that of labour versus capital.

Unfortunately I was not able to keep Drago in any kind of therapy, but the disability agency informed me that the addition of a medication that helped reduce his impulsivity and increase his tolerance towards frustration allowed him to hold down a job in a car wash. Sure, it wasn't a dream job, but it gave him some structure and purpose. I doubt he took much notice of my interpretations around his fatherlessness, but I'm confident his anger towards racial groups was tempered once he was able to maintain some kind of employment.

Darryl on the other hand was a difficult but eventual success story. Instead of projecting his rage outwards he was able to see that his own failures of communication and regulating mood were major contributors to why his life had gone the way it had. The moral, individual dimension of his problems became more apparent, mediated through the secular process of therapy and psychiatric medications. He managed to keep his new partner, just, and he had initiated contact with his children after many years.

# 7

# MUJAHIDEEN TO MCMANSIONS

Treating refugees is deeply humbling. If ever there was an appropriate context to the notion of First World problems, it is assessing an African refugee at the beginning of the day. I was in a fluster after spilling a coffee on a maroon woolen jumper, bought from a luxury store situated on the Champs Elysees in Paris. Not usually one for high fashion, I wanted to show off what I hoped to be a new, more stylishly presented phase of my career.

Alas, as is the tendency of my clumsy self, in an attempt to juggle the morning coffee in the car's cup holder, a burst of flat white erupted from the styrofoam container to scar my hopes for a more fashionable me. I swore loudly while attempting to change lanes, examining the brown stain like I would a flesh wound.

A half hour of podcasts, tolls and traffic jams later, I arrived at my practice to see the waiting room full of a large, extended family of Africans. I take great pride in being able to tell the difference among Asians: Sri-Lankans and South Indians tended to be darker with flatter noses; Koreans had rounder faces and usually more muscular builds; Pakistanis looked fair, almost Arab; Cantonese Chinese were quick to differentiate themselves from mainlanders, preferring Hong Kong as the answer to where they were from and not China. But with Africans, I had little idea. They were a new group in terms of migration to Australia. Nor had I travelled to that part of the world given its relative inaccessibility.

On this morning there was a family of five ready to enter my rooms. The patient was the father, named Henok. Tall and lanky, his skin was a glistening, jet black that gave his eyes an extra glow. He was the definition of exotic and I felt positively albino in comparison.

His three children remained in the waiting room, playing games on phones much like any other kids, and Henok was accompanied by his equally tall wife, Hedisti. The letter from his family doctor asked me to review the medications he was taking for a likely psychotic illness, which meant at some stage his thoughts had lost touch with reality.

Henok was softly spoken and his wife took the lead in the telling the history. They were Eritreans and arrived almost a decade earlier as refugees from a civil war with Ethiopia. While Henok had been able to maintain odd jobs in factories and briefly in an abattoir, he was now suffering vivid nightmares waking him from sleep and preventing him from functioning. Hedisti wept relating how her husband screamed at the children and no longer had any interest in intimacy.

As Henok began to engage with me, horrific details of his experience in the civil war emerged. Much of his extended family was hacked to death, including a brother killed in front of his eyes with a machete. He told me this matter-of-factly, his facial expression barely changing. Dreams of such an event had re-emerged for him in the past few months. He woke from sleep in a sweat, sometimes hitting his wife in the middle of the night while screaming in agitation. The children avoided him and preferred to go to the local park with their uncle.

My role was to increase his anti-psychotic medications, which were designed to tranquillise him, stabilise his moods and dampen the over-activity of some of his thoughts, based on the fundamental changes in the way he perceived threats around him. I expected a strong cultural dimension to the consultation, perhaps a belief in spirits or a view that he might be cursed or a deep shame about his symptoms. Instead his wife was clear in her understanding of the notion of post-traumatic stress disorder, referring to nightmares and avoidance behaviours.

Henok feared the crowds in shopping centres because they triggered memories of murderous mobs. To be fair, some shoppers are ready to kill for Boxing Day bargains and may wield handbags and manchester as weapons, but his fears were testament to the power of painful memories, especially those associated with imminent death. But when I asked Henok about what his mental illness was, he frowned, bowed his head ever so slightly and said, "crazy head".

Hedisti was clearly sophisticated. In her forties and dressed in a tightly hugging, floral dress, she carried herself with a great dignity. The family was educated in Eritrea, although Henok only had the opportunity to complete high school before war erupted.

They had functioned well until recently. The trigger seemed to be greater difficulty finding new work for Henok and strong financial pressures to manage the children. He lacked meaningful skills and the factory work he relied on was dwindling. He was facing similar pressures to many of my working class patients struggling to get a leg up in the post-manufacturing, advanced, service economies of the West. Hedisti tentatively raised the future prospect of the disability pension but didn't dwell on it, her shame at the prospect of becoming dependent palpable.

Here was Henok, a man who had endured brutal civil war, the

murder of much of his family, many years in an Ethiopian refugee camp and travel halfway across the world beginning to fall apart as his provider role was feeling under threat in the suburbs of western Sydney. His mind, wanting to make connections to other periods in his life as a way to help him cope, comes up instead with his war experience, a woefully inadequate analogy to his current circumstances.

A fragment of a smile emerged when I suggested a small increase in his medications may alleviate a great deal of his suffering, but he had little interest in revisiting the war or what the return of the nightmares might mean. No one wants to revisit traumatic memories over and over, but it was also indicative of a trend I see in ethnic patients in their reluctance to engage psychologically, a relative disinterest in psycho-babble.

In his book on cross-cultural mental health, *Crazy Like Us: The Globalization of the American Psyche*, anthropologist Ethan Watters travels the world looking at how Western concepts of mental illness were transforming the experience of madness in traditional cultures. He writes:

> The ideas we export often have at their heart a particularly American brand of hyper-introspection – a penchant for "psychologizing" daily existence. These ideas remain deeply influenced by the Cartesian split between the mind and the body, the Freudian duality between the conscious and unconscious, as well as the many self-help philosophies and schools of therapy that have encouraged Americans to separate the health of the individual from the health of the group.

But in my experience, unlike Watters, the uptake of mental health in most ethnic groups was limited to the physical view of mental illness that was more acceptable and reduced stigma. It was also more consistent with the physical symptoms patients experienced

– dizziness, headache, abdominal pain – as a way of expressing their emotional distress. But the psychologising side – the Woody Allen, sit on a couch side – of mental health was not attractive at all and too culturally foreign. The unique, interior life as some kind of pointer to an individual truth was too inaccessible.

This had significance because the non-medical side was often the link between individual agency, personality and the emotional symptoms. Learning how one coped was the key to modifying it for the better. But for the many patients who lacked what is called psychological mindedness, most commonly those with limited education or from ethnic groups, their ability to modify their symptoms struck significant limitations.

I found refugees interesting when examining how quickly ethnic groups adopted Western practices for they were often the most different. Like lower socio-economic groups, their relatively rapid uptake of mental health language was a pointer to how psychologised modern society had become. Patients like Henok accepted medications to treat illness but were resistant to trying to understand any deeper meaning associated with the symptoms, unless it was culturally mediated.

An insight Watters makes in his book, however, is that traditional ways other cultures may make meaning through spirits or rituals are being downgraded and replaced with a disease model of mental illness. Much like traditional cultures were swept away with Western-borne diseases or fatty foods in the heyday of European colonialism – they were thrust on them so quickly their physiologies and cultures were not able to adapt – refugees were representatives of ethnic groups adopting Western practices but in unsophisticated forms. They struggled to maintain any kind of individual agency when confronted with mental illness.

Unlike skilled migrants who for the most part had already worked in multinational corporations, were from middle class backgrounds and envisaged themselves as global citizens, the average refugee was exceptionally relieved to have received migration to an advanced country like Australia that offered free education and health services, not to mention a strong welfare safety net.

A study conducted in 2015 by the Sydney Refugee Health Service in conjunction with the University of Western Sydney, measured several hundred patients who presented to the service with mental health problems. They were primarily Iraqi refugees. The study was borne from the conflicting data surrounding refugee mental health and whether the patients actually improved while receiving treatment or were likely to decline when faced with the challenges of resettlement.

The patients' symptoms were measured when they first presented versus several years later. A key finding was that despite them accessing treatment, the measures of their symptoms were often worse as time progressed, presenting real difficulties for refugee and welfare services.

The nurse unit manager heading up the service, Sandy Eagar, hypothesised that refugees arrived to Australia with a great sense of optimism and purpose and this was reflected in their psychological state. But within a few years, despite receiving appropriate treatment and the variety of government services on offer, the combination of traumatic histories and the challenges of surviving in Australian suburbia took their toll. Ms Eagar was reticent when asked about their prospects surrounding integration, but noted that the largest group of recent arrivals from Iraq or Syria were deeply disturbed when they arrived to the service, their tales of starving, dead children or the murder of their relatives overwhelming to some of the service's workers.

But another possible conclusion from the study about poor

outcomes of many refugees with regards to their mental health have overlaps with my patient Henok, whose vulnerabilities became more exposed when interfaced with the rapid changes in political economy. Integrating the modern refugee in an economy that increasingly lacks jobs for unskilled workers, particularly those with limited English skills, is more difficult. It is a far cry from the influx of Mediterranean migrants that arrived post-war to take their place in enormous job creation schemes like the Snowy Mountains project or the wide availability of manufacturing and unskilled jobs that Vietnamese refugees had access to. While it is true the children of refugees are more likely to progress up the social ladder, it is also true the first generation are likely to become dependent upon welfare.

Another patient I treated illustrates how refugees may rapidly absorb some Western norms, but the notion of the interior life can still be illusory, unappealing or just plain inaccessible. When I received the file with the name of Adam Hancroft, I did not expect to meet the child of Afghan, Hazara refugees. Adam was a young man in his twenties, olive skinned with plucked eyebrows, silk shirt and a striped pink tie. He loosened his tie as he entered my room and sat down as if to signal he was ready to shed a psychological load. Unlike most patients, he was eager to begin and leaned towards me, making penetrating eye contact.

"I don't feel nothing, doctor. Talking to people is like talking to rocks," he said, raising his hands as though pleading.

I needed to reorient the interview.

"I can see you're distressed and eager for help, Adam. Perhaps start with how your problems are affecting your life," I said.

Adam said he didn't have big problems, just that he woke almost mute, occasionally had panic attacks and struggled to stay on any medications. Despite being in great distress, he was simultaneously eager to minimise his difficulties.

"I'm curious how you came to have a name like Adam," I asked.

He changed his name after becoming an adult, feeling that his original name, Mohammed Sarabi, might hinder his dreams of worldly success. The name came from a video game character.

"But it's not relevant to what's going on," he countered, after a brief answer, irritated.

"Everything's relevant in this game, Adam," I suggested with a smile, "...but go on."

Adam had recently married a girl from the local Hazara community and started a new job in disability services. He had seen another doctor but couldn't tolerate the several anti-depressants he had tried, mainly due to sexual side effects. Zoloft, Prozac, Effexor, Lexapro – he had tried all the common ones.

"I just got married. It's just too embarrassing if I can't have sex or, you know, come," he said. A common side effect of anti-depressants was delayed ejaculation, something that was also quite useful for people who tended to be premature.

Adam spent much of his early life in a Pakistani refugee camp before coming to Australia when he was ten years old, as part of the United Nations allotment. He was the second of four children. His father was an engineer who'd had a construction business in Kabul.

"We didn't come in a boat," he underlined. "We're legit."

I found it interesting that he, an Afghan refugee, might have the belief that those who came by boat were ripping off the system, but I didn't pursue it.

While Adam appeared to cope well in school, he struggled in his first job as a public servant, having filed a successful bullying claim.

"I felt intimidated. The manager spoke to me so loudly," Adam explained, shaking his head.

In this initial appointment with Adam, several warning signs came to my mind. His difficulties staying on tablets and also his original doctor told me it was likely he struggled to form and maintain relationships. This was usually related to what is known as "attachment", or effectively, the bonds we make as a baby with our mother. I knew the chances of him returning to further appointments were low and I would need to make extra efforts to form a trusting, effective relationship. His poor compliance with medications was also a reflection of this. While the side effects were real, sticking to tablets was also a relationship and often an extension of the bonds formed with the prescriber.

His wife, Shahada, attended a further appointment and wept at Adam's difficulties in showing tenderness, unable to touch her outside the sex act, during which he was often rough. He was so desperate to connect, it seemed, that he did so in a clumsy and rough way. In the midst of his difficulties he was determined to believe that if only the right medications were prescribed, he could be rid of his problems. Then he could resume his path to some kind of career nirvana, fuelled by the power of positive thinking transmitted via his bookshelf stacked with Tony Robbins and Tim Ferriss self-help manuals. He had inherited some aspects of psychological thinking, but it was of the unreflective kind aimed at fulfilling immediate desires through positive affirmation.

In between our appointments he sent emails outlining what he felt was too slow a recovery. Email has transformed therapy for it allows another, often more introspective mode of communication.

Here is one Adam sent:

> You see my depression isn't the usual in that I try to go about my daily life as normal as I can, I guess it's called the walking or smiling depression. Behind it all though, I'm crippled with self-doubt, negative thoughts, anxiety and constant feeling of sadness.
>
> I put on a brave face to people and go about daily life as best I can, but behind the mask I am suffering. I never really feel like I fit in anywhere and it's like I have to try to act to be happy in every day situations. It's hard to describe, but it's almost like I'm standing behind my shadow. I always look at other people and wonder what it's like to be just happy.

His emails show a much greater depth than he was able to communicate during consultations, but the email also came after several appointments and after we built a stronger relationship. It was satisfying that he was beginning to examine his internal experience.

In later appointments I discovered his mother suffered a serious post-natal depression while living in Afghanistan. Adam did not initially see it as relevant given she had recovered since migrating but it was like a "cha-ching" sound for me, a key clue as to how his early life bonding may have been disrupted. If living in in the midst of war and waiting years for a refugee outcome wasn't enough, a serious case of depression almost certainly affected how Adam, who was Mohammed at birth, may have thrived. I couldn't help thinking that his bullying claim in the public service may have more to do with his perceptions of mistreatment and innate low self-esteem.

When it came to the sudden collision of refugees and Western concepts of mental illness, there was no better or more politically heated example than detention centres for asylum seekers. My esteemed colleague and former Australian of the Year, Professor Patrick McGorry, called detention centres "factories for mental illness". Multiple studies have shown that a large proportion of asylum seekers satisfy the criteria for depressive or anxiety disorders.

Yet it always amazed me that a set of people who had survived amid conflict zones with their lives in danger, able to travel by land, air and sea to the other side of the world, fell in a heap when a fence was placed around them, in spite of them being sheltered and fed.

The community leader, breast cancer survivor and former Liberal Party candidate Dai Le speaks of her time in a refugee camp as unremarkable. "We just played. We didn't know it was bad."

United Nations reports about refugee camps around the world, all of which would make Australian detention centres in places like Villawood look like the Hilton, never detail outbreaks of self-harm or epidemics of mental illness. Physical health problems exist aplenty and it is possible mental health is a lower priority in such settings, but it is also true the expectations of the refugees are far different. And nor is it an unusual space influenced by fractured domestic politics and a refugee advocacy industry baying for government blood. There is no such context in UN camps.

Detention centres illustrate one of the great weaknesses of mental health diagnosis, masterfully exposed by a 2008 book called *The Loss of Sadness*, which describes how context has been removed from mental illness. In Professors Wakefield and Horwitz's account, they outline how cause has been removed from diagnosing mental illness in favour of a list of symptoms. What we call depression is often an appropriate reaction to loss or the continual pursuit of an unreachable goal.

This is an apt description for many of the asylum seekers who take enormous risks for the potential reward of permanent residency in Australia. When these expectations are dashed, it is not surprising any ensuing rage or frustration would tick the boxes for mental illness.

Likewise the self-harm outbreaks are also subject to an unusual set of incentives not present in other UN refugee camps. Self-harm in detention centres is similar to the contagion effect that can occur in school playgrounds, a little bit like children spreading viruses. They can be genuine attempts at suicide, a release of overwhelming tension or malingering, where there is a potential gain from feigning an act. The reason for self-harm can also be a combination of these and not entirely conscious.

There is no question that asylum seekers are in great distress with few outlets to communicate it, but it is also irresponsible to discard the possibility that an unusual set of incentives for migration may skew behaviour.

But fault cannot be placed on the asylum seekers. Why wouldn't you try for migration when it could mean you improve the situation of countless members of your family? Imagine a lifetime of free health and education services and, where necessary, welfare benefits that would be the equivalent to the highest paid jobs in the asylum seekers' countries of origin.

The inequalities and luck of birth are unjust, and inequality is the biggest driver of migration flows, including that of refugees. Migration experts such as the late solicitor David Bitel, who was closely aligned to the Left of politics and a vocal supporter of the UN Refugee Convention, told me that coming by boat was just too easy to rort and was dominated by middle class Iranians. I interviewed him before he died about his experience of refugees and mental health. Bitel undertook the first worldwide case on behalf of a gay refugee in the early 1990s but was also accused of encouraging some asylum seekers to fake their homosexuality. I had worked with him on writing psychiatric reports for Bangladeshi asylum seekers.

Whether the asylum seekers are in detention or living in the community it is the uncertainty of living in a traumatic limbo which is intolerable. That is the prime contributor to the distress of asylum seekers. The detention part of their circumstances is overplayed as the main traumatic factor.

What many people don't understand about the anger towards boat people is that it is expressed not just by white people perceived to be racists but also by skilled migrants. Migrants from non-English speaking countries who come to Australia through the rigorous skilled migration program go to enormous lengths and spend exorbitant amounts of money. Those who come as students toil for years in low paid work before receiving permanent residency. Their families often sell their assets to pay for the tuition.

While all migrants have sympathy for the desire to access a better life, many also experience resentment when they see boat people trying to undercut a system that demands a certain level of qualifications and gain migration. I too have this feeling and think about scores of my relatives in Bangladesh tirelessly and expensively attempting to conquer the necessary courses and bureaucracy to gain entry through the Australian points system. All of them are aware of people smugglers and the prospect of coming by boat. Much of the asylum seeker debate falls into the category of the identifiable victim, which in this case is someone capable of paying a large amount of money to smugglers.

But psychological studies also show that refugees can trigger in all of us unconscious associations with the notion of trauma, extreme experiences that expose us to fears of death, hopelessness and exile. These unpleasant feelings can be intolerable and our impulse can be to turn away.

My interest in refugee health is in the uptake of psychological concepts and what forces shape it. Detention centres illustrate how Western contexts and incentives can align to rapidly and dramatically shift the emotional experience and its communication among refugees.

Another Afghan refugee patient I treated fought in the mujahideen, the precursor to Al-Qaeda. His name was Farhad and he had fathered several children before arriving in Australia with his family. In his early sixties, he had led an extraordinary life. Broad shouldered, muscular and with a brown curly moustache I imagined him carrying a Kalashnikov over his arm while patrolling the mountains for the Soviet enemy. He was proud of defending his country from outside forces but preferred to keep quiet about it. He said his children knew little about his time fighting for the mujahideen. But his dignified, physical presence in my consulting rooms gave me a clue as to why no colonial power has been able to conquer Afghanistan for centuries.

His daughter accompanied him to his appointments, an attractive young woman studying to be a pharmacist who also functioned as the Farsi interpreter. Farhad was suffering from worsening headaches and beginning to have dreams of his time in the war. They had been dormant for decades. His GP thought his symptoms resembled post-traumatic stress. Farhad told a story about holding his friend in his arms on a ledge of a hill as he slowly died from the wounds of a Russian grenade. He thought he could hear the folk song he sang to his dying friend in his dreams.

Our interviews were brief as I could obtain little more about his symptoms other than the headache and how he could no longer drive for any length of time before he became distressed. In Kabul he worked as a taxi driver for almost two decades and he was not affected by psychological symptoms, but here he was, much like my Eritrean patient Henok, undone by McMansion suburbia and metropolis drudgery.

Farhad's anxieties were financial and a concern that he couldn't support his children before they married. Notably he was planning his daughter's wedding soon after she graduated. His lack of English limited his ability to become a local taxi driver and the business of mixed Afghan stores selling spices, transferring money and functioning as a community hub was becoming a mature market. His daughter said there were almost seven of them within a ten kilometre radius of where they lived. Unless Farhad could attract a market as an after-dinner speaker at Afghan parties and tell his stories about fighting as a mujahideen solider, his options were sorely limited.

I had little choice other than to place him on a disability pension. Thankfully his children were thriving. I was not convinced he was suffering from a post-traumatic stress disorder. His disturbing dreams were likely to be a reflection of his broader anxieties around the family's future security.

There are an enormous number of refugees thriving in Australia and they reflect a different type of migrant in the mix. They're more likely to take risks, be entrepreneurial and their success stories are incredible. But they are also more likely to fall in a heap with greater odds stacked against them. They reflect the extremes of the migration story, from Frank Lowy to Man Haron Monis.

My patient Adam surprised me and was becoming far more insightful into his psychological frailties. He was very eager, perhaps too eager, sometimes stifling a gentle disclosure of his inner life. He was bright and educated, which gave him an advantage. His wife also became involved, which helped illuminate how his symptoms stifled core relationships. But he remains one of my most challenging patients, recently divulging that if we were living in America he would access a gun and end his life. Each session is draining, his suffering a palpable weight in the room.

I continued to treat Henok and enjoyed seeing a slow recovery. His nightmares began to settle and, encouraged by his dynamic wife, the couple started a business exporting used car parts into Africa. A contact of theirs in Ethiopia then distributed them to street markets in the capital. I was intrigued by the twists of globalisation I heard of in my consulting rooms but suspected it was Hedisti who was doing most of the work. Henok was helping with unloading goods and interacting with customers.

I still think of them when I spill coffee on my clothes.

# 8

# THE TROUBLE WITH TEENAGERS

I had never heard of a school counsellor until I was studying psychiatry. When I was in Year 11 in high school I was invited to have one session with a careers advisor. At the time, I was doing well in economics and the adviser suggested I work for a bank or in policy. I was mortified that she thought I might suit such a job and questioned my entire persona. I was proving unsuccessful in projecting a smart-arse, larrikin vibe if the careers person thought I should become an accountant.

But her advice was the original role of a school counsellor, which involved giving guidance usually in terms of academic subjects or future job choice. In parallel with our more psychologised times, this role has become an indispensable aspect of the therapeutic necessities of the modern school.

Much like employers have counsellors attached to employee assistance programs, educational institutions have psychologists working specifically for schools. They are now the first contact for many kids whose psychological vulnerabilities are exposed amid the social and performance pressures of school. Despite their role being aimed at assessment and referral, in practice many become the key therapist in a child's life.

We sure could have used them when I was in school. Bullying

was rife and barely questioned. In primary school I remember a lovely girl being called Smelly Ray, solely because it rhymed with her Christian name, Kelly. There was no objective evidence that she had any kind of unusual or unpleasant odour. We even made up a song beginning with the line, "Smelly, smelly Rae", lyrics that Bob Dylan would have been proud of. I barely knew her but found myself joining in, partly because I had my own fears that I smelt of curry and wanted to deflect any possible attention on body odour.

The harassment went on for almost a year. I have no memory of any kind of formal intervention from teachers. The belief back then was this kind of behaviour was relatively harmless and that it would pass. I suspect in most cases this was true, but I see my share of psychiatric patients who give histories of horrific bullying at school and its impact remains lifelong, contributing to a brittle self-image. Often it emerges in workplace disputes where the worker feels unfairly treated but in fact their history of bullying sensitises them to misinterpreting criticism or feedback as intimidation.

At my high school, teachers sometimes joined in. A boy in our year was caught masturbating at home by another student—he surprised him by walking in through the back gate. A teenage boy masturbating is about as newsworthy as the sun rising in the east, but the problem was that he got caught. Despite the friend professing to keep it secret, the entire school knew about it within days. During a school assembly that week, the PE teacher began a speech by yelling "tugger" into the microphone, to the hysterical laughter of every one of us. From all reports the boy turned out fine but I wasn't surprised that he made little effort to attend high school reunions.

None of this kind of behaviour would be acceptable today. The dark side is that many teachers complain that their role has never involved a greater focus on managing emotional and behavioural issues. My observations from assessing compensation cases involving school teachers is there is a heightened sensitivity around bullying. It is often used as a weapon in playgrounds and in the battlegrounds of office politics. But the rise of school counsellors represents a significant advance in the mental health of children, especially when such diagnoses have become so endemic.

One of my most interesting adolescent patients who illustrates many of the challenges was Jane, a teenage girl of East Asian background. She was sent to me by her psychologist because of her problem in attending school. Jane was in Year 8 in a selective school. She complained of terrible headaches and hearing voices telling her to hurt herself when going to sleep at night. She stuttered when interacting with other pupils at school, but not at home. On the days she did attend school she would return home, play video games and engage in social media where one boy harassed her to "go kill herself". Her Korean parents could not make any sense of what was happening to their daughter, and the situation was made worse by her father's employment being in Seoul. He would fly back and forth every few weeks.

When Jane attended her first appointment she was dressed in a Mickey Mouse T-shirt and her hair was in pigtails. Her manner of dress was an immediate sign that she was regressed, which means she was becoming more childlike under distress. Under an experience of trauma, even adults can start sucking their thumb or wetting the bed.

I asked her how she felt about coming to see me.

"Are you gonna put me on anti-depressants?" she enquired in a soft, shaky voice. "I've read about them, you know – fluoxetine is good for kids, isn't it?"

I understood immediately that she was very bright, probably

perfectionist, and had researched her treatment at great length. Her childlike passivity was also a clue that she might have trouble asserting herself with others and perhaps experience others who were a little forthright or blunt as attacking her.

"We might, Jane, but I need to understand you a little better," I said. "Tell me about school."

She initially sat next to her mother on a small couch in the corner of my consulting room before I asked her to sit alone on a different chair. In teenage years our challenge is to start separating from our parents and put a greater focus on bonding and belonging with peers. Parents of ethnic origin don't place the same emphasis on encouraging autonomy and separation within their kids as Western parents and I wondered if Jane was clingy with her mother. I did discover that Jane had suffered separation anxiety as a child and her mother had had a difficult pregnancy and complicated delivery.

I was confident that the psychologist had referred Jane because she was hearing voices and, because of this, psychotic illnesses like schizophrenia had to be excluded. In the appointment it became clear that she was unlikely to suffer such a terrible diagnosis for it seemed to only occur at night when she was alone with her thoughts. I started her on tranquilisers, suggested group therapy and explained to the family that her headaches and voices where like mini nervous breakdowns. There was every chance she would improve slowly, but it was destined to be a hard slog.

There has been an explosion in disability provisions provided for mental health diagnoses for high school students in recent years. The trend is Australia wide, but the use of provisions is skewed heavily to the students of elite private schools. For some schools such as Sydney's St Andrew's Catholic School, the figures revealed a whopping one in three students sitting for the Higher School Certificate had registered themselves for a disability provision.

While school administrators suggested many parents chose the school because it prided itself on catering to those with a disability, when the proportion of people diagnosed with a mental illness reaches such levels, the notion of illness loses its meaning. It becomes virtually the norm.

The principal of St Andrew's Cathedral school, Dr John Collier, offered a revealing quote in the *Daily Telegraph* when asked about the issue. "Teenagers are less resilient than they were a generation ago, and more likely to fold and seek professional assistance." he said.

Likewise the prestigious SCEGGS Darlinghurst has upwards of one in five students registered for disability provisions each year. SCEGGS's headmistress, Jenny Allum, explained that these provisions cover a full range of needs – from the ability to take jelly beans in the exam room for diabetic students, different coloured paper or different sized text for those with some visual issues, use of a scribe for those who can't write with their usual hand, through to rest breaks for those suffering some forms of anxiety or other mental health issues.

But in response to Dr Collier's comment about the diminished resilience in teenagers these days, Ms Allum told me that she wasn't surprised by the rise in diagnoses and that expectations and pressures on high school students had never been higher. "the pressure on kids these days to have perfect CVs - great grades, a range of leadership opportunities, and demonstration of community service is significant, even before they start work. Competition to get into a good university and the emphasis on the HSC and the Tertiary Entrance Rank is significant. It is tough being a teenager these days!"

Nor are the privileges insubstantial, varying from scheduled breaks, scribes or sitting in an adjacent room to protect some anxious kids from the shock of facing large groups. Those students unable to sit examinations are given a mark commensurate with their performance in assignments throughout the school term.

It is true that the better off were more likely to access specialist mental health services. Ethnic groups and the less well off may not consider such distress as abnormal or see their problems through the lens of mental health. Girls were over represented, just as they are in anxiety disorders as adults. It is difficult not to see the perfectionistic personality traits of many such girls combined with the high expectations of their parents and schools being the critical triggers. But this can hardly be new.

The statistics bear out the considerable increase in psychiatric diagnoses among the young. A 2015 government study revealed one in seven children aged between four and seventeen qualified for a mental diagnosis in the past twelve months, meaning over half a million kids suffered a mental illness for the year studied. The most common diagnoses were attention deficit disorder and anxiety disorders, particularly social phobia.

The explosion in self harm is noticeable in my work. Figures across the Western world illustrate a marked increase in measured self-harm, but nobody can say for sure whether this is related to measurement, sufferers more willing to volunteer the information or it becoming a more common expression of emotional distress.

When asked this question in an interview aired on the BBC, Cambridge child psychiatrist and academic Dr Dickon Bevington stated anecdotally there was much evidence teenagers were in greater distress but scientific data wasn't available to confirm this. Two key areas he identified as having clearly increased in incidence included self-harm and abnormal eating behaviours – both in males and females.

Dr John Collier's view that teenagers were less resilient today had some figures to support it. He qualifies his statement saying his views were not based on any kind of quantitative study but observations over a forty-year career, including working in disadvantaged areas such as Campbelltown in outer Sydney.

"I haven't seen the level of decompensation before where students collapse in a heap and are admitted into hospital for psychological reasons just before an assessment or examination," he says. He cites the decline of what he calls meta-narratives such as religion leaving many teenagers out in the cold when attempting to acquire a sense of purpose. Filling this gap is a shallow search for happiness that he interprets as lacking any attachment to any broader structure of meaning.

Dr Collier's views are strongly based in his religious outlook and faith. He correctly identifies that in such a highly diverse society, which is arguably now post-religious, there is no binding scaffolding that can give people a strong collective identity. This problem extends well beyond teenagers but can be significant for adolescents because their search for belonging is profound.

But I do not think staunch atheists are more likely to collapse psychologically, although in times of crisis religious faith can provide solace. In today's social circumstances, those who become actively religious are a minority group and often find belonging in religion because of their difficulties integrating with mainstream life. This is particularly the case in Muslim teenagers but is prevalent across the social spectrum. I have assessed several adolescent patients who benefited greatly from joining charismatic groups such as Hillsong. Their black and white thinking patterns were cushioned and channelled in healthy directions.

But school counsellors are more circumspect about whether teenagers are any less resilient today than in the past. While most who work in the public sector cannot be quoted freely, the majority I speak to while treating kids tell me there is no clear evidence that children are any less resilient and that the very concept of resilience is in rapid flux.

The senior counsellors are in agreement, however, that the combination of more fragmented families, working parents, a poorer tolerance of failure among kids and a greater focus on material success are contributors to why our children seem more brittle in the face of adversity. This outlook identifies the prospect of higher expectations as being a possible contributor to adolescent strain, especially in a secular meritocracy where we are all fed the idea of infinite social mobility.

The counsellors who worked in more affluent areas also told me that there was pressure upon teachers and schools not to miss diagnoses such as autism, which attracted extra resources. This is certain to be a key contributor to the phenomenal increase in autism rates in recent decades. Threats of legal action or what one counsellor called "going Ministerial" in reference to complaints to the Department of Education were not uncommon and a pointer to the environment the modern teacher must navigate.

With regards to the greater pressures for all of us to be incredibly amazing and successful, American studies at least bear some of this out, showing when teenagers were asked if becoming rich was a priority, those responding yes tripled from 25% to 75% in three decades.

I am regularly asked to fill out the disability provision forms, as I did with my patient Jane, although she was several years away from her final examinations. The children and their families are in great distress and are not doing anything wrong. They are within their rights. There is usually an extra urgency when the time of examinations draws near.

While the majority of presentations are around anxiety disorders, usually perfectionistic kids having panic attacks when faced with the prospect of failing or feeling overwhelmed to the point where only self-harm relieves their despair, there is also a less discussed but growing proportion of families who present believing their children suffer attention deficit and may benefit from Ritalin. This is an interesting aspect of mental health where treatment can verge towards performance enhancement.

The project of success and self-improvement, when channelled through the children, reaches a social zenith in late high school. The intense meritocracy of the modern age becomes apparent through the distress seen in children. It is no wonder they are called canaries in the mine.

An unspoken aspect of these trends is that middle class, predominantly white children from elite private schools are competing with highly driven, goal-focused children in public selective schools who are now consistently outperforming them for university entrance marks. The trend is most rampant in Sydney and Melbourne but it is spreading, heightened by the fact that the dominant migration is coming from countries like India and China. A patient of mine said there was only one Caucasian student in his year of high school at the top selective school, James Ruse Agricultural High, and even that heritage was one-quarter Russian.

The children of immigrants bring a desperation that is at odds with the stereotype of the relaxed, larrikin Australian. Globalisation in Australia brings with it a degree of Asianisation, at least in education. For example, last year in New South Wales, public selective schools represented the top eight in Higher School Certificate rankings before the first private schools, Abbotsleigh and Sydney Grammar, showed up in ninth and tenth places respectively.

What these results represent are fundamentally different views of human nature clashing through our school system. The predominantly Asian parents of children in public selective schools, as popularised through the notion of Tiger Mums, are unashamedly elitist, see children as resilient and able to cope with pressure, view intense competition as a social reality and are sceptical of the notion of self-esteem separate from actual achievement. There is conflict when their children assert their individuality, be it through extracurricular activities that are not considered academic by their parents or through social interests at odds with conformity.

Public selective schools are often disparaged as mark factories by headmasters, who claim that the schools place little emphasis on building broad-thinking skills. I remember an explicit aim at my high school was a British notion of the Renaissance man, one who might carry his violin case to rugby training before completing his homework in advanced physics in the evening. There is also the contested idea of how to transmit values in schools, one that attracts heated controversy, such as when the program Safe Schools was released with its emphasis on the fluidity of gender.

This building of broader interests is one area many Asian parents underestimate the importance of in parallel with their reduced emphasis on social and communication skills. The importance of these "soft" skills are pronounced in service economies like Australia's, where technical skills can be outsourced but creativity is highly prized. Israeli philosopher Yuval Harari identifies the capacity for storytelling and building myths as the single most important characteristic that allowed humans to develop so significantly in comparison to other primates. These social skills are not rewarded to the same extent in more conformist, hierarchical Asian countries, but such attitudes are in the process of rapid change.

Jane's parents were aware of this potential to hot-house their children. They paid for tutoring in preparation for selective school entry but also encouraged her to pursue her interests in playing piano. The striving instinct was hardly unusual when parents were making significant sacrifices. Jane's mother said if Jane didn't achieve entry into a selective school, they would have saved obsessively and paid for a private school or moved to an area where they could be confident of a good, local public school.

"If there was one thing I would change about the education system today, it would be to rethink public selective schools," said Head of School Jenny Allum. "They have been the death of the local, public, comprehensive school. More than anything else, the existence of selective schools has established a hierarchy of government schools, and this has meant that the local comprehensive school is perceived as 'inferior'. In leagues tables (something Ms Allum abhors), it appears that the best schools are selective schools, followed by independent schools, followed by local comprehensive schools. This is such an issue for our society. Of course if you pick the really brightest students for a selective school, that school will do well in any Leagues Tables constructed. It doesn't mean that those schools are any better than the local comprehensive school – just that they select their students on academic ability."

Dr John Collier believes that while poverty is the key contributor to poor educational outcomes in the developing world, he identified affluence as exerting a dragging effect on children in our society, describing many kids of the rich as 'languid' and lacking the same drive for upward mobility that immigrant children invariably have. He also states that a minority of parents use private schools to outsource their responsibility for the leadership role of parenting, citing one example of a parent employing their own personal assistant to deal with any phone calls relating to the schooling of their children. If only. I'd be curious to know what might be the title on the business card of such a person; perhaps educational relationships expert or parenting assistant.

In elite schools such as Geelong and Knox Grammar there has been a parallel growth in the notion of "positive psychology". This philosophy is drawn from Harvard psychologist Martin Seligman's ideas around harnessing and developing our core attributes and focusing on positive emotions. While there is much to commend Seligman's theories, its popularisation as depicted on Geelong Grammar's website, where it states the school's philosophy encourages students in "feeling good and doing good" has its limitations and potentially does harm in stigmatising difficult emotions and reducing the individual's ability to manage them. It's difficult not to see some of these trends as a kind of branding exercise for some private schools, a symptom perhaps of having too much money to spend.

A focus on positive emotions is rooted on a humanistic philosophy popularised in the theories of psychologist Carl Rogers. The whole world of self-help and motivational literature has its roots in such a philosophy. The philosophy has the most significant psychological influence in the modern conversation and pervades many organisations and institutions. The optimism of modern America is infused with this view of human nature. The movements of self-esteem and pride helped propel the civil rights movements of the 1960s and 70s. It helped correct the messages of inferiority that many minority groups such as blacks and women had absorbed for centuries.

The belief is that religious thinkers and Freud placed too much emphasis on the dark side of human nature, our sinfulness and our capacity of aggression and selfishness. According to humanistic philosophy, this has repressed our true, authentic selves, as represented by our feelings. As Zac Efron sings in High School Musical 2, "I wanna listen to my own heart talking/I need to count on myself instead/The answers are all inside of me."

The emphasis on feelings is magnified at a time when most people in the Western world have hollowed out identities and are no longer tied to a religious view of the world. Humans are innately social and constructive according to thinkers like Rogers and Abraham Maslow, who coined the term "self actualization".

But the emphasis on getting in touch with our positive emotions arguably stigmatises the more difficult, unpleasant emotions that are a staple of day-to-day life. The most common mental health problems children and teenagers experience are an inability to tolerate such negative emotions, which is understandable if the dominant message is that our positive emotions and shiny optimism are the keys to fulfilment.

School counsellors also observe that kids had fewer problem-solving abilities in difficult situations and more commonly found unpleasant emotions intolerable.

Colleagues in psychiatry, such as the profession's representative for adolescent mental health issues, Dr Nick Kowalenko, said at a practical level the rise in adolescent self-harm was often a direct result of parents not being around and not being able to contain their children's emotions at difficult times. But he agreed concepts such as self-esteem and positive psychology had their limitations.

Positive psychology often descends into a bastardisation of the notion of self-esteem, which itself has considerable question marks as a useful concept. In 2005, a landmark *Scientific American* article, titled "Exploding the Self Esteem Myth", examined multiple studies looking at the benefits of self-reported esteem and found little correlation with long-term academic or social success.

There is clearly a class dimension to the problems of high school students. Another headmaster who had also worked in the education system for thirty years is Mr Malcolm Hurley. His work has exclusively been in the most disadvantaged areas of western Sydney. When I asked him about teenage resilience, the key difference he cites is the social and family breakdown endemic among his pupils. Students regularly disappear for days, often living from the house of their friends or relatives. Divorce, drugs and teenage pregnancy are rampant, particularly among his pupils from housing commission estates or Aboriginal and Islander backgrounds.

Mr. Hurley also noted that the living arrangements of many of the parents were organised to maximise potential welfare payments such as carer pensions or Centrelink benefits. The difference to the students in elite schools is the markedly different expectations around educational results and social fragmentation. But despite the obvious social problems, the kids were unlikely to present to mental health, let alone apply for disability provisions.

Mr Hurley also observed the greater focus on bullying and while this was positive in protecting a small subset of vulnerable, passive kids, it also encouraged a less cohesive workplace and playground with smears of bullying, racism or even abuse used as a weapon with no fear of penalty for false accusations.

Along with statistics and the observations of experts there is also some biological evidence that support the hypothesis that youth today find life more challenging, despite living in the most prosperous and peaceful times. As government studies have illustrated, anxiety disorders are prevalent in this stage of the life cycle and neuroscience confirms this by noting the parts of the brain that are well developed in late teens include the amygdala, which regulates fear, and the circuits of the brain that control reward.

Meanwhile, the parts that are responsible for calm reasoning in the pre-frontal cortex, don't fully develop until age twenty five. This combination means teenagers are both more likely to be anxious but also more likely to enjoy the potential rewards of taking risks, an unusual and problematic combination. And, of course, the rational, problem-solving part of the brain is relatively weak, as any adult trying to parent a teenager knows.

Another aspect of biology that has changed is the steady reduction in the age of menarche, the time when girls begin to menstruate. The age has been gradually reducing over the last century from about seventeen years old to now just below thirteen. It's believed to be due to improved nutrition and the reduction of infection. It is now equivalent to the age which our hunter gatherer ancestors became fertile.

But the psychological implication is that girls living in the West, and increasingly in the more prosperous sections of Asia and South America, are sexually mature well before they have reached any kind of emotional maturity, adding another layer of complexity to their psychological demands. Menarche may have been a factor in my patient Jane, who had her first period only six months before seeing me. This sexual awakening may have sensitised her to the boy's rude online remarks, being more self-conscious of her sexual attractiveness.

Anthropologists and social scientists have made reference to traditional societies that had a communal ritual, like an initiation or a rite, to facilitate the process from immaturity to maturity. Few such processes exist formally in Western society, other than perhaps a twenty-first birthday party or a hard drinking session with male friends and relatives on turning eighteen. Self-harm may signify an attempt to reclaim such rituals, especially when you consider some kind of laceration or regulated harm often play a role in traditional initiation rituals.

The psychiatrist and coiner of the term 'identity crisis', Erik Erikson, argued that the very notion of adolescence emerged with industrialisation. This brought a greater focus on the nuclear family as opposed to clan and community that agrarian social organisation naturally lent itself to. As child labour was stamped out, a period of life emerged that allowed for a more structured emotional and intellectual development while the child was still under parental authority. While Romeo and Juliet are sometimes held up as the quintessential idealist, emotional teenagers, the notion of adolescence didn't exist in Shakespearean times.

The arrival of a distinct new life stage also came with a greater distribution of responsibility for the socialisation of young people. The social transformation that came with industrialisation brought with it an ambiguity. Prior social functions carried out within the family such as economics, social control, education and religion are outsourced to specialised institutions, most notably schools and sometimes churches and sports clubs. The alternative institutions have their own, distinct rules and regulations and permit different levels of autonomy and participation.

If the nuclear family was appropriate for a time when manufacturing and traditional industry was the basis for our economies, it is worth asking whether a different model of the family is necessary in the information age. What might the networked family look like? Perhaps just as female biology is beginning to have similarities with our hunter-gatherer ancestors, the information age may allow for a smoother use of clans and communities in child rearing. Arguably, this is already happening among the small proportion of families raised in the kinship models of same-sex parents. Whatever you think of gay marriage, homosexual parents are usually so anxious about their children not getting a healthy range of input they are more assertive in self-organising a clan model of child rearing.

My primary place of work is in a private hospital in western Sydney, a beautifully designed, sprawling sanctuary with manicured gardens and edgy artwork on the walls of the corridors. Small rooms fill with patients attending group sessions on everything from managing sleep, preparing to go home to understanding the side effects of their medication. The therapeutic complex can be observed in all its glory with mental health nurses distributing medications, psychologists huddling patients into interview rooms, art and music therapists and even a gardening expert running horticultural groups.

Those patients who have private health insurance arrive furtive and reluctant, fearful that they may be booking themselves into an insane asylum along the lines of 'One Flew Over the Cuckoo's Nest', but usually leave chuffed and upbeat. Those who are transferred from public psychiatry wards are usually the most relieved, having spent time in relatively decrepit buildings surrounded by the most unwell patients with schizophrenia or drug-related psychosis.

The hospital has one of the few private adolescent wards in New South Wales, and desperate families come from all over the country seeking treatment for their teenage kids. The presentations tend to have consistent themes. Psychiatric diagnoses are grey at the best of times, but during this time of life they have even less validity, because the diagnosis is likely to be different when the patient is seen further down the track.

It is rare the kids themselves initiate the admission to hospital, a program that encompasses a combination of group and individual therapy for three weeks. Group therapy is difficult to access within the public system, a major gap given the importance of social anxiety within the adolescent stage. The referrers are usually school counsellors or psychologists.

The most common reason for referral is teenagers who are no longer able to attend or function at school. This is known as school refusal and is regarded as an emergency in the field. The kids are usually having panic attacks, sometimes self-harming, and might have begun using drugs, most commonly marijuana as a way of self-medicating their fear and agitation. Parents are distraught but often have their own histories. It may be a mother who suffers an anxiety or depressive disorder or a father who cannot manage his anger and who the child finds intimidating or critical. These are stereotypes, but they tend to be more common scenarios.

My patient Jane fitted some of these stereotypes. I encouraged her to attend the group therapy in our hospital, which is useful for social anxiety. Groups are powerful in recreating a social world and we tend to respond to others in such therapeutic groups much the same way we might to people in the real world. Jane was so fearful that what she might say would be perceived as uninteresting or silly that she stuttered at the beginning of each sentence. The fear was not so dissimilar to the fear of dying, except it was anticipating a social death. This is particularly paramount in our society where a sparkling, gregarious personality is prized, a cue to how we might have reached a point where shyness was allowed to be medicalised.

Jane was a bookish girl and she taught me that the Japanese version of social anxiety, which was called taijin kyofusho, involved a fear that one's own inappropriate social interactions might embarrass or upset other people, indicating the stronger collective, hierarchical context of Japan.

Dealing with modern teenagers can feel like encountering an alien species. Perhaps it was always thus, but technology does highlight the gap. I have had adolescent patients who wanted to conduct interviews through text messages, so frightened were they of having to interact with a flesh and blood human unfiltered through any kind of digital interface, and my unpredictable habits of asking questions and writing in a file.

Stilted language, a penchant for storming out of the room, mostly when parents detail their symptoms and its effect on the family, and pervasive distractibility are norms, so much so that I think attention deficit is a relatively normal adaptive response for teenagers and their world of screens and social media interaction. One-on-one interviews combined with involvement from parents is hardly adequate and there is now a greater requirement to understand their social media behaviour and their lives in the world of chat rooms and multi-player online games. Several patients I have treated have had their own online groups glorifying self harm, sometimes sharing videos of themselves cutting to be shared with their friends.

I don't believe social media is the cause of many pathologies, but it can magnify pre-existing problems such as bullying or normalise pathological behaviour such as self harm. Its greatest effect is in magnifying fears of comparison, forever seeing other people's greatest hits and curated images of apparently perfect lives. When this aspect of social media is seen in parallel with our focus on self fulfilment and the importance of projecting a performed, authentic outer self, we can start understanding why adolescents may never have had it more difficult, at least psychologically.

The smartphone is one of the most powerful democratising devices in history, but as former Kings School headmaster Dr Tim Hawkes said to me, teenagers are not the best people to harness it: "They're P plate minds with full access to V8 technologies, sometimes a recipe for disaster." It is adolescents and their intense urge to belong and heightened sensitivities around the prospects of social humiliation that make them the most vulnerable.

One of the first requirements of the hospital program is a digital detoxification for 48 hours, which can send some patients into outright hysterics or a decompensation into panic. Observing such reactions might be amusing if they weren't so tragic and they illustrate the dark side of technology and how it is used as a crutch for the vulnerable. While it is most likely Western civilisation was already on a path towards atomisation, narcissism and anxiety well before the influence of the internet, working at a private psychiatric hospital makes me wonder if it accelerated the process.

In her book *Alone Together*, MIT social scientist and psychoanalyst Sherry Turkle outlines how many teenagers no longer answer the telephone, finding its immediacy disturbing, whereas Facebook posts and text messages can be honed to give the impression of spontaneity. Her studies of teenagers and their interactions with technology are pertinent to my job and, like her, I can't help think of the implications to our humanity if the way we communicate is altered so rapidly.

But teenagers' underlying desires and needs have not changed. They want to feel loved and they want to belong to something. The pain of not belonging is never so strongly felt as it is in adolescence even if their tempestuosity appears to signify selfishness and a pathological individualism.

I am especially sensitised given I have two daughters not far from entering high school and the full onslaught of teenage social and technological complexity. While parents can place strict boundaries on activities outside the house, the boundless world of the internet can be a boon for teenage rebellion and experimentation. There is considerable evidence that, just as social leaders like headmaster John Collier has stated, teenagers today do have unique pressures heightened in technology, parental attitudes and the prevailing culture.

# 9

# BRICK LANE IN LAKEMBA

I'm too lazy and comfortable to do aid work in poor countries, despite professing my aim to do so as a medical student. Law students dream of saving political prisoners from despotic governments before opting for careers reorganizing tax structures for corporations. Almost every medical student initially dreams of working in the amorphous, hazy idea of the Third World, which for some was equivalent to working away from the inner city.

But I made an attempt while doing my compulsory elective during university. While several of my colleagues were hard at work putting together dissertations on topics like 'Diving Injuries in the Caribbean Island of Aruba' or 'Respiratory Ailments Encountered while Trekking in the Himalayas' I threw myself into a cholera hospital in Bangladesh. It was horrific, tens of people lined up across each floor, lying on thin foam mattresses linked to drips for dehydration. It looked post-apocalyptic but was mundane for the Dhaka based institution famous for inventing a saline solution to treat diarrhoeal diseases.

Within a week my skin was turning yellow and I had succumbed to a digestive illness. The most likely culprit was unfiltered water used to wash a salad I shared with a relative at an otherwise posh restaurant. It wasn't until I returned to Australia having shed ten kilograms that I was tested at a laboratory to discover I had contracted Hepatitis E.

The infectious diseases professor assessing my case was positively ecstatic and called me several times to arrange appointments. Feeling chuffed that he was so interested in my diarrhoeal project I soon learnt that Bangladesh was one of only three countries in the world, along with Bolivia and Peru, where the virus even existed. Professor Kotsiou was interested in me as a post infectious specimen and not for my elective project. He liked me for my body and not my brains.

I have since opted to scratch my developing world itch by seeing patients who had migrated from there, from refugees to newly arrived migrants. As virtually the only qualified Bangladeshi psychiatrist in the city, a common presentation are Bangladeshis who otherwise would never consider their problems varying from headaches to excessive washing as psychological in nature.

A memorable case that illustrates many of the issues in such a group was a woman called Farzana who arrived to my rooms accompanied by her bearded husband.

He began the story and painted a picture of Farzana, living in a stifling hot tiny flat in Lakemba, putting their two year old daughter in her cot, and perpetually fulfilling the rituals of wudu – purification. First she washes her hands three times, each time reciting the Arabic phrase 'subhana-alla'. Then she moves on to a gentle rinse of her forearms to her elbows – also three times. Finally her face, mouth and back of the neck.

In a cracking voice dripping with concern Shakil said Farzana sat cross legged on the brown, cotton prayer mat she aligned with Mecca. She always checked the compass application on her smartphone to make sure the direction was correct, before praying once more.

I had learnt to pray as a child. I rarely did now but I could imagine Farzana engaged in the choreography of bending down to place her forehead on the mat, kneeling to recite a particular section of the prayer and standing to repeat key verses. She heard the call to prayer from the neighbouring mosque as a notice for another imminent prayer.

The problem was that twenty minutes later, she began her purification again.

Farzana was typical of so many of my patients who present for psychiatric services but have little interest in receiving them. Their suffering does not feel like illness, but just the mundane drudgery of conscious living laced with a particularly intense emotional suffering.

Those from ethnic or lower socioeconomic groups rarely see any kind of suffering through the lens of mental illness, but are more likely to be referred when other specialists have investigated and ruled out the possibility of a physical diagnosis.

This is especially true when people present in couples: the person with the greatest needs may not be the person who initiated the session. As well, presenting as a couple may encourage a patient to disguise their real need so the other person takes more responsibility. A person might present as seeking to save the relationship, when really they want permission and a safe way to end it. Or vice versa.

Shakil leaned forward, concerned, while Farzana hung back, furtive and not making eye contact. Her nose was pierced with a thin, golden ring and her head covered with a portion of her blue sari, some platted locks of her dark hair visible. I noticed some light calluses on her hands, but my observations were interrupted by Shakil.

"I want to help her, but don't know how," he said, leaning forward in his cream coloured taxi driver uniform, with its embroidered logo on the breast pocket, his booming voice filing the room. Although speaking in an Indian accent, occasional words such as 'mate' or 'sure' were pronounced with an exaggerated Australian twang. I imagined him speaking to his passengers trying to mimic them.

He was loud and seemed overbearing and controlling. Farzana cowered in his presence. I wondered if it was he who was in need of help but had no insight or desire for self examination.

He lamented how he did not receive much in the way of welcomes when he returned home or that food wasn't prepared for him when he arrived. At the beginning of their marriage, a union he said was arranged through the extended family, Farzana dutifully arranged bowls of curried meat, dahl and boiled rice in the cramped kitchen before placing them before the seated Shakil on the coffee table. She even had bowls of mango chutney and green chillis cut in halves to be enjoyed as accompaniments. But these days when Shakil returned late at night from his usual shift, their daughter was asleep and his wife was deep in prayer. There would be nothing to eat but leftovers.

In spite of my initial wariness towards Shakil, I thought his disappointment was appropriate in what appeared like a traditional marriage from within a strict, Islamic cultural background. The preparation, delivery and joint eating of meals was the most common communication of affection in a traditional culture. But problems rarely just surfaced and I thought it may signal a tension in the relationship that existed before Farzana's decline.

The nature of their union, an arranged marriage via rural Bangladesh, suddenly transported into suburban Sydney, already marked their relationship as complicated. Newly married, isolated women from ethnic cultural backgrounds were a common presentation in my practice, particularly given western Sydney was one of the more diverse melting pots in the world.

Beauty or brains have traditionally been seen as the paths towards social mobility, often through marriage, but mass migration has added another fast track option, the spousal visa to a wealthy country like Australia.

I escaped an arranged marriage. Despite my parents not being religious, they had an expectation I would marry a Bangladeshi despite having migrated to Australia decades ago. My father was ready to place an advertisement in a Bangladeshi newspaper in search of a bride even after I had been with my partner, and now wife, for several years.

"Bangladeshi Doctor living in Australia wants beautiful, well-educated woman to marry. Has Permanent Visa and Satellite Television."

Prior to that he considered a union with the daughter of a corrupt former Bangladeshi politician who had fled to Australia after being exposed for siphoning off foreign aid into his own Swiss bank account. He sold off thousands of tonnes of sugar and came to be known as Sugar Zafar, but because he hailed from the same region as my father, he was deemed to be a friend. Zafar's daughter was more suitable than a white girl in my parents' eyes, at least for a time.

Agreeing to such a marriage was a nod of respect to continuity and tradition, particularly in the face of the considerable sacrifice in terms of cultural and family disruption that elders felt through migration. While my parents did not entirely share it, there was a view among many migrants that they would simply live the same way they always did after arriving in Australia, but just do so more prosperously. It was only through the children, and to some extent the workplace, that their practices and outlooks were challenged.

Arranged marriage seems ridiculous to most of us now, but we forget romantic marriage is a relatively new concept and is still an unfinished revolution in most parts of the world. In countries like India and Bangladesh ninety percent marriages are still arranged and many young adults are satisfied with this arrangement.

The historian Stephanie Coontz in her book *Marriage: A History* writes "(marriage) had as much to do with getting good in-laws and increasing one's labour force as it did with finding a lifetime companion." The idea of marrying for love was considered a serious threat to the social order. Order has traditionally been valued more greatly than freedom.

Even in the 1990s, newlywed Russians at the height of glasnost rated love as the fifth priority among the top ten reasons for marriage and a third of all French women claimed that their male partners weren't romantic enough. This was discouraging. If the French with their poetry and obscure philosophical references weren't considered romantic, my prospects for points were limited with wilting roses and tickets to emerging, indy theatre.

I had some family friends explain to me the strategic importance of an arranged marriage. By marrying someone approved by my parents I would cement their status through their friendship and family network. But as an added bonus there would be an entirely new family that would have access to the sponsorship points that would allow potential migration opportunities to Australia. When you add the remittance payments in Australian dollars, arranged marriage was its own foreign aid program. It is also one of the strongest indicators of a resistance to integrate.

Measures of arranged marriage are not easily found in Australia, but in Britain South Asian groups had the lowest intermarriage rates of any ethnic group. It was particularly high among Muslims from Pakistan and Bangladesh. There was a social class component, given South Asians emigrated to the United Kingdom often as unskilled immigrants and had a harder time rising up the social ladder. The lower levels of education also meant they set up ghettoes such as those in the WhiteChapel area of London. They returned to their ancestral villages when it was time for the children to marry.

In a book over a decade ago, British Bangladeshi author Monica Ali wrote a novel *Brick Lane* about the challenges of a newly married Bangladeshi woman, having migrated from a village, who found herself in a stifling union with a much older, misogynistic, unsophisticated husband. The book outlines her attempts at exerting some individuality within such a framework. The main character begins a clandestine romance with another Bangladeshi man in the East End.

The book alludes to something that was called the *Begum syndrome*, a condition that Bangladeshi mothers were said to suffer amid the relative poverty and disadvantage of their situation. They visited their doctor complaining of "burning in my head" and "life pressure". Researchers concluded that their talk of "beesh", which was the Bengali word for poison, was a kind of somatisation and internalisation of their cramped dwellings and limited resources. The so called syndrome was an anxiety disorder transmitted through the culturally appropriate expression of physical symptoms.

Like *Brick Lane* in London, Sydney also had its suburbs that were effectively holding areas, temporary zones for migrants who had not yet settled, whose lives are defined primarily by their past – theirs or their parents – but who want to grab the future. Lakemba was one such suburb, often the initial point for whatever the latest wave of migrants were in much the same way Brick Lane housed post war Jewish arrivals before the Bangladeshis.

In the past decade Lakemba was less the home of the Lebanese and increasingly the hunting ground of sub Saharan Africans, Pakistanis and Bangladeshis. They set up their restaurants, supermarkets that offered money transfer services and they congregated at dinner parties and the local mosque.

I regularly treated women like Farzana, who lived in Lakemba. When I turned my attention to her during my initial assessment, there were calluses on her hand, unusual for modern women living amid the abundance of domestic, household appliances. I remember visiting Bangladesh as a child and marveling at village women toiling for hours applying soap on clothes, rubbing them fiercely with their hands mimicking a washing machine. The relief of completing this task was usually met with the call of the kitchen and another few hours preparing food from scratch over a clay stove and firewood. The calluses on Farzana's hands were more likely to signal excessive washing or rubbing as a repetitive behaviour.

I wondered whether any tension among the couple was exacerbated by their different status. In Bangladesh a high status woman like Farzana would never marry a taxi driver. But Australian citizenship elevated the negotiating power of otherwise ordinary men, sometimes creating marked mismatches. Other women like Farzana I had treated often arrived in Australia only to realise the man they had married was not in fact a 'transportation executive' or 'hospitality entrepreneur' as they may have spruiked in the marriage negotiations, but in fact a taxi driver or even a kitchen hand. The negotiations usually took place through phone calls between relatives and exchange of documents such as work resumes and birth certificates. But marriage fraud had reached epidemic proportions such that many families in South Asia were increasingly suspicious of overseas suitors.

There was also greater pressure on the relationship between spouses in modern marriages, whereas in the past such unions were cushioned by interactions with large, extended families. Even among couples choosing their spouses, psychological studies show we are increasingly reliant on our spouses as ties to the number of close friends and other networks have dwindled. As a result, even with the greater tolerance and expectation of compromise that those entering arranged marriages inevitably had, conflicts are harder to endure.

Farzana's husband had not touted himself as a transportation executive, but nor did he advertise his relative poverty in a place like Sydney. He arrived in Australia on a tourist visa in the mid 1990s but overstayed. I saw little point in prying about how he obtained citizenship, but knew there were a host of techniques varying from temporary, sham marriages to employer sponsorship. My own family helped illegal immigrants struggling for money and accommodation when I was a child in western Sydney.

Another kind of problematic, arranged marriage that arises are when children are too scared to stand up to the authority of their parents and agree to unions they have little interest in. The poor partners arrive only to find that their new spouse has in fact a boyfriend or girlfriend not acceptable to the conservative, ethnic parents. One patient of mine was even told to sleep in a different room a few nights a week while his spouse made love to her pre-existing, personal trainer boyfriend. The parents were oblivious to the arrangement.

It seems inconceivable that anybody would put up with this situation but the new, imported spouse often has a significant disadvantage in that their migration status depends upon the marriage with the Australian citizen. Consequently, they feel powerless and unable to stand up for themselves, especially when their family back home is depending upon them for the marriage to work.

This happens to both men and women. They present to me because one way they can retain their migration status is if some kind of abuse occurs and they can argue they suffered a diagnosable mental condition, then the government may clear them to live in Australia in spite of their marriage failing. It's quite an obscure loophole in our rules but one that migration experts are all too aware of.

A common player in upholding abuse against new partners is the mother in law, particularly when the migrating spouse is a female. A divorce or failed marriage is devastating to family prestige and to be avoided at all costs for strict families, even those based in Australia.

According to a 2013 ruling in the Indian Supreme Court, a significant proportion of the several thousand dowry related deaths in India each year are overseen or ordered by the mothers in law. Such abuse was described by the presiding judge as reflecting "an emotional numbness in society".

Dr Manjula O'Connor, a psychiatrist based in Melbourne, specialises in domestic violence within Indian communities. She has recommended anti dowry legislation be implemented in Australia, a clear example of illiberal ethnic traditions playing out in the suburbs. She emailed this quote about the potential risks in arranged marriages.

> An arranged marriage is a collision of hopes and ideals. He dreams of a traditional wife who will take care of his cultural needs, bring up his children in traditional manner and someone easy to control. She dreams freedom, autonomy, control over her life, great job, great life style.

Dr O'Connor's views had resonance in Farzana's case. I would need to see Farzana alone before asking about any prospect of abuse.

"How is the marriage?" I asked matter-of-factly, applying the doctor's power to instantly access the most intimate aspects of patient's lives.

Shakil was not taken aback. He said their marriage had been strained while Farzana's symptoms were worsening, particularly as Shakil was forced to reduce his hours working as a taxi driver because of her behaviour. There were also occasions when she had not properly fed their daughter or prepared lunches for day care. On one occasion Farzana was so ensconced in prayer that their daughter, Aisha, had not been picked up at child care and Shakil received a phone call from the manager of the centre.

"This was very embarrassing," he said, emphasising it further by adding the Bengali word for shame, lajja. The word struck me as particularly strong, and highlighted his sense of humiliation.

The unusually powerful response from Shakil made me wonder about topics less likely to be raised, like drug and alcohol use. This was unlikely in devout Muslims, but abuse of prescription medications or even chewing the betel nut leaf were more common. This was a bitter tasting nut wrapped in a leaf, mixed with tobacco or other spices. Much like kava for Pacific Islanders its consumption might be a way of reminding Farzana of home. I also knew the codeine in strong cough medicine was a drug of addiction in Bangladesh, particularly amongst the youth. It was the poor man's heroin. But Shakil assured me that there was no such problem. Farzana gave me a look of disappointment that I had even considered such a possibility. She narrowed her dark eyes and furrowed her brow.

I asked Shakil to leave so as to interview Farzana alone. As well as feeling more comfortable talking about intimate details, people often reveal non-verbal markers that gave important information about the relationship when they are assessed alone. A teenager may suddenly uncross her legs when her mother leaves the room, and in doing so reveal scars related to cutting and self-harm. A woman may more clearly expose bruises associated with domestic violence as soon as her partner steps out. Realising this, the abusive partner in a violent relationship is often particularly reluctant to leave their spouse alone in the consultation room. But when I asked Shakil, he simply looked towards Farzana who nodded and so he left us alone.

I asked Farzana about her life in Bangladesh. Newly arrived women, particularly after arranged marriages, are at risk of sudden isolation, especially after losing the support of extended families in their ancestral lands. I imagined my own mother arriving with my father decades ago, in a similar position, terrified of the outside world. She still complained there were no decent spice stores in the 1980s and that new arrivals had it easy now.

During my handful of visits to Bangladesh, I can barely remember a time when I had been alone, such was the sheer density of people, both indoors and outside. The idea of loneliness was an anathema, met with bemusement. Conformity, suffocation and the prospect of being crushed by crowds was more of a reality.

"I am a good student but had few friends," Farzana begun. As was typical of people from her background she began with her academic status when asked about her childhood, whereas Westerners related it in terms of being happy or sad.

"Poro-shona was important in our home. Baba, Ma were teachers," she said, noting the importance of education. She only had a younger brother, which was an unusually small family. I asked whether the mother had fertility difficulties or perhaps there were problems in the marriage. Farzana didn't know.

The place of religion was relatively minor in their households, in spite of them being surrounded by great religiosity within the community. Farzana said her mother often spoke about how as a child, women wearing burqas and men growing long beards were barely visible, but it seemed to increase during Farzana's lifetime. The region of Noakhali, where they lived, situated in the south eastern corner of the country not far from Burma, was particularly known for its conservatism. The local mullah was powerful, commanding as much authority as the Member of Parliament. This marked Farzana's family as particularly modern and progressive, which may have explained their small size.

"I hoped my husband would be more modern too, but he is not," she said, in a sharper tone. Her statement pierced the room like an arrow. I recognised its significance. In her softer way, she was expressing profound rage. I didn't pursue it but made sure to acknowledge it. She continued with tales from her development.

Her parents were both teachers in the local district high school in the southern part of the Bangladesh. It was near to the birthplace of my own parents, adjacent the Indian border. There was a significant presence of the Islamic party Jamaat-e-Islam in their district adjacent the Bay of Bengal, and they created a degree of resentment in Farzana's parents. She told me that a Jamaat office bearer once chided a teenage school girl for flicking her hair too seductively. Farzana remembered her father having a verbal conflict with a man parading a long, henna stained beard. She worried about her father, but the scuffle settled. Farzana noticed days later that the girl in question started wearing a head scarf to school.

Farzana also described the period when her maternal grandfather died. She was barely ten years old and remembered her mother soaking a tea towel with water and rubbing his forehead several times a day. Children were kept at arm's length from sick relatives, the belief being they were not mature enough to see such suffering. Her grandfather, who she described as having an especially long, henna stained beard in his final years, couldn't swallow for months.

I enquired whether he suffered gastric or oesophageal cancer, but Farzana wasn't sure. When he died after a tortuous few months, she remembered the household being transformed into a prayer sanctuary. They were flooded with grieving relatives, cupping their hands together to pray, a practice known as dua, usually while holding prayer beads. The beads numbered ninety nine, corresponding to the number of names given to God in the Koran.

Farzana expressed surprise to see her mother suddenly involved in the religious fanfare, which she didn't understand at the time, given their family appeared virtually atheist. Her mother said that things would be clearer when she grew up, that it was impossible to process death without some kind of religion.

My psychologically sensitive ears pricked up.

"Why do you think you remember this Farzana? What does it mean?" I asked, thinking the sudden religiosity of her mother may be related to Farzana's own sudden religiosity. Her response was a surprise.

"I think about death more often," she said, making direct eye contact. "I worry about my daughter dying, maybe from asthma or being kidnapped."

"Does she have serious asthma?"

"No, but she was in hospital as a child for a breathing problem. I know it's silly."

"Who else are you worried about dying?"

"My mother and father in Bangladesh. They are getting old and I am not there to look after them. I feel guilty at times."

"Do you worry about your husband?"

"Aktoo," which was Bengali for 'a little'. "But he is stronger than me and can work for long."

While death anxiety was in the background for many patients, this didn't seem to be what drove Farzana's pathology, which she soon confirmed when she began to talk about an unusual, undiagnosed abdominal pain as a teenager.

It was put down to "gastric", which is a term used to describe acid reflux in the stomach. Farzana touched her abdomen while describing it and pulled a sad face identifying it as distressing. It was unlikely the notion of irritable bowel syndrome was considered in Bangladesh. There is a host of terms in medicine for when medical science can not give clear answers, such as non-specific pneumonitis, idiopathic colitis or anxiety disorder not otherwise specified. Irritable bowel is in that category, a pain that had no associated physical pathology attached. The symptoms are common in my ethnic patients, along with headache or dizziness, and was often related to anxiety where the culture didn't provide other outlets to communicate it. The condition confirmed for me that Farzana had a prior history of anxiety that wasn't identified as such.

I examined Farzana's hands and had a closer look at the early signs of calluses from the repeated washing. She also exhibited a tiny bump in her forehead from the praying, which even had a word in Arabic 'zebibah', translated as raisin. Her mother did not sound anxious, but Farzana said that her mother suffered a bout of tuberculosis soon after giving birth. I wondered whether her anxiety was triggered by some disturbance in the initial bonding to her mother.

At this stage, I raised a critical aspect of the encounter. Did Farzana think there was a problem?

"My husband is very worried, I know," she said, becoming more relaxed and engaged. She leaned forward in her chair. "He thinks I can be a better mother and wife."

"And you?"

She nodded sheepishly. She did want help and could see possible benefits for her, but there was a degree of reluctance. I asked her to expand about her marriage.

"I thought coming to Australia, I would be part of a more modern society, but it's like going back to the village living with Shakil sometimes." she spoke more rapidly and was holding back tears. "I thought I would make him happier if I was more religious, like his family."

While Muslim immigrants often became more religious on arrival to Western countries as a kind of defence to perceived hostility from the dominant culture or nostalgia for the ancestral home, Farzana's newfound religiosity seemed to be an unconscious way of seeking approval from her traditional husband.

She said the call to prayer audible from the local mosque calmed her. She described her compulsion to pray, relating her ritual, from the purification to the repeated bending, standing and kneeling. For completeness, Farzana showed me the compass application she used to align her prayer mat on her smartphone.

She revealed the home screen with a photo of her daughter, Aisha, smiling at the camera with red ribbons in her hair. Farzana bowed her head in guilt and shame when I commented how beautiful her daughter was.

I brought Shakil back into the room, who anxiously looked towards Farzana before sitting back on the couch. "What do you think bhai?" he addressed me more familiarly as 'brother'.

I asked them both whether Farzana engaged in other rituals such checking locks.

"Yes, she goes round and round the house closing the windows, even on the hottest days." Shakil answered instantly, with a hint of frustration. I imagined him returning after a twelve hour shift driving a taxi across Sydney, dealing with drunks, party goers and office workers only to be trapped in a stuffy, overheated tiny flat.

I turned to Farzana, who sheepishly referred to the linen in the bathroom.

"I re-arrange the towels after each prayer, so they are perfectly symmetrical, no loose or uneven folds," she said, eliciting initial surprise from Shakil judging from the squinting of his eyes, before he nodded his head and made eye contact with his wife in a moment of shared insight.

I diagnosed Farzana with obsessive compulsive disorder, given her repeated rituals and thoughts that if she did not wash her hands, something terrible would happen, such as her daughter might die of some kind of illness. This was typical of OCD, which went beyond merely wanting to be clean or safe, but was usually related to an intrusive, automatic thought that if not responded to with an action, caused overwhelming distress. It was her version of the Begum syndrome the Bangladeshi women in London's Brick Lane suffered decades ago.

But I wondered if Farzana's retreat into prayer was in some way an identification with her mother, who responded to the grandfather's death with sudden religiosity. There was the possibility she was experiencing her life in Australia as a kind of loss and was in a state of grief, particularly as her parents aged. While they were not yet frail and sick, Farzana imagined it as imminent. Most people from other cultures view themselves as relational beings, inextricably linked to clans and places. Farzana may have been experiencing a psychological decline due to feeling a split with her parents and a disruption of her role as a daughter, further heightened by being a mother to a girl herself.

There was also the elephant in the room of a strained, marital relationship and the mismatched expectations of both parties, which could not be sorted during this consultation.

The treatment was relatively straight forward in some respects-the prescription of an anti-depressant. I wrote her a script, and asked to see them again in a few weeks.

The couple did not return for over a month, and then Farzana reported that the improvement in her symptoms was only marginal, which was not a surprise. When I explained that she had been on a minimal dosage, they became more positive. Shakil pointed out that even on this low dose, there had been a noticeable reduction in Farzana's anxiety and praying.

Encouraged, she reported that her relationship with her parents were improving too. I discovered that Farzana had been so ashamed that she had not mentioned anything to her parents and avoided speaking to them. The reduction in her obsessional praying as a result of her reduced anxiety about cleanliness had also led to more contact with her mother, perhaps diluting her sense of dislocation.

I was concerned that Farzana remained socially isolated but ironically, when her general practitioner looked into women's groups in the area, though there was a specific one aimed at Bangladeshi women it was at the mosque and based around reading Koranic verses together. We decided that Farzana's need for social connectedness outweighed the risk of increased religiosity.

I asked Shakil during our second appointment about Farzana's belief that he was too traditional in outlook.

"No, no, no. I want my wife to work. I am not backward at all. I don't know why she thinks that," he protested. "But we also have 'shomaan' to consider in the community." 'Sho-maan' was a word for honour.

"What do you mean by shomaan?" I asked, although having a pretty good idea. My father made reference to it when he worried whether my sister and I might do something untoward, like join a bikie gang, inject heroin or not go to university, possibilities that were generally seen as equally dishonourable.

"Look, I am not a mean man, but when she first arrived to Australia, she was wearing expensive dresses and silk scarves and skirts. People talk. You know our community," he said. "But it is better than praying so much."

I understood that the expensive dresses were seen as negative, a symbol perhaps of a flashier, more Western minded woman.

I doubled her dose of anti-depressant. Farzana was praying only a few times a day when I saw her again, as compared to the twenty or thirty times previously. She also brought me a gift of gulab jamuns, balls of fried dough glistening in sugary syrup packed into a clear, plastic container. I was interested whether her religious beliefs had changed as her devotion to its rituals waned.

"No, I believe in Allah. Of course, I do," she said, a little insulted. "But praying all the time does not make me a better Muslim and does affect me being a mother and wife." She was more confident and started wearing skirts and T-shirts to appointments. From Shakil's history, I recognised this was closer to her norm. She was more engaged in the surroundings and made jokes about the hospital patients visible through the window.

"Doctor Sahib Tanveer, you are lucky I did not come into hospital." she said, pointing to a patient with tattoos and dyed, blue hair. "I think I would have coloured my hair blue. Hehe." Her giggle and grin was seductive and alluring. I checked myself.

"How did the praying and washing help?" I enquired.

"I just feel dirty, when I was worrying and worrying. I was not a good wife or mother, I think," Farzana answered. Her reports were consistent with obsessional rituals often being related to excessive or even superstitious ideas surrounding purity; I was still not sure if her acting religious was a way of hiding her washing rituals or an attempt to impress her husband.

Shakil was circumspect when I brought him in briefly at the end of sessions. He was pleased that they were beginning to socialise again, but concerned that some of their friends gossiped that Farzana was becoming too modern and Westernised, no longer wearing a headscarf and buying fashionable clothes. It seemed that he was indeed traditional in his outlook and that Farzana was not religiously minded at all. The episode had shifted the dynamics of the relationship, so that Farzana felt more in control of her destiny.

I had not seen them since but received a message from Shakil that Farzana was running a rapidly expanding family day care service and even learning to drive, overcoming a long term fear. I hoped the new income stream might dilute any of Shakil's concerns about Farzana becoming too modern.

# 10

# Why Addiction Is Like A Love Affair

I seldom get nervous before seeing patients, but I felt an unusual anxiety before seeing Lynne. She had been referred to me by a high school friend, now a medical specialist, who told me Lynne was a beautiful young woman from a highly regarded Orthodox Jewish family. Hers was not a demographic associated with western Sydney, but Lynne was prepared to travel to consult with me. She was disappointed in her relationship with an elderly Jewish psychiatrist, a practitioner she had been seeing for several years since developing a worsening prescription drug addiction with opiates and benzodiazepines like Xanax.

I had progressed from growing up in an environment where there was considerable antipathy and outright loathing for Jews to developing a strong affection for them as an adult. I went from hearing about global Jewish conspiracies intent on dominating the world during Bangladeshi dinner parties to attending bar mitzvahs at high school.

While working as a junior doctor, I supplemented my income

by making house calls in an area of Sydney with a large Jewish population. I became a member of the Hakoah Club after treating the manager's wife and grew to love matzo dumplings. I regularly attended several households of Orthodox Jews. Their families were large and their possessions sparse. I also remembered from university that Ashkenazi Jews were susceptible to genetic blood disorders. I admired Jewish groups for managing tradition with modernity, being able to compete at the highest levels of business, technology and science, yet still keeping a foot in the synagogue and the Torah.

My initial encounter with Lynne was awkward.

"You don't support Hamas, do you?" she said, making firm eye contact. "They're terrorists, you know."

This was an unusual beginning to a patient interaction, but also brought a smile to my face. If Lynne could be so direct so early I was optimistic she might be a good candidate for sophisticated input.

Flanked by a husband in Orthodox Jewish uniform – black hat, long beard, black suit and white buttoned shirt – I felt a tinge of excitement that Lynne would be a stimulating, albeit demanding and difficult, patient. In religious terms we were like a duo – the lapsed Muslim and the Orthodox Jew. If ever there was a Jewish science it was that of psychology.

She was a year younger than me and despite her being a little overweight, much of her status as an Hasidic beauty queen was still apparent: chiselled features, long frizzy hair and an alluring cheekiness. Our sessions were lively. They inevitably involved at least one reference to the Lynne of yesteryear, the vivacious version of her in late teens and early university life. She repeatedly told a story about giving speeches to hundreds of people and being coveted by multiple men. She lamented that she no longer felt desired by her husband, Joseph, who was too focused on religious matters and the death of his father. Joseph was observing a mourning period of eleven months of the Hebrew calendar.

I admitted Lynne into the clinic to reduce her use of codeine and Valium medications. The clinic was an intensive program of group therapy and individual counseling to help patients withdraw from drugs or overcome a psychological crisis.

It became clear that her migraine pain had strong psychological origins for it worsened when we reduced her Valium yet we had not altered her codeine. Valium does not treat pain but she expressed the panic and anxiety of withdrawal in the form of physical aches. There was an anguish visible in a tortured, twisted facial expression and her body shook irregularly as tears rolled down her cheeks.

Lynne had experienced migraines since she was a teenager and was able to manage them with over the counter tablets. They worsened in her late twenties and the pain spread throughout her body. In the past she had been diagnosed with fibromyalgia, which described a diffuse pain that didn't have a clear physical origin. It was when the pain worsened that she was introduced to codeine and benzodiazepines. She rapidly developed an addiction. Now the addiction threatened her marriage and was causing havoc with their four children, one of which was being schooled in Israel. She struggled to prepare meals, attend to guests and was terrified of attending synagogue.

Her childhood history contained potential clues about what kind of psychic wound lay beneath the addiction. She grew up in a large family and experienced her mother as cold and distant. She was sure her mother also suffered a mental illness but didn't care for treatment. I knew there was a greater potential for sexual abuse in conservative communities with strict segregation of sexuality. Lynne did allude to some unwanted, uncomfortable encounters with relatives when she was a teenager but didn't think they affected her. But she hinted that her sexual attractiveness was seen as a potential problem amongst her pious family and a marriage to another Orthodox Jew, Joseph, was organised in her early twenties.

Another patient of mine, Jeremy, developed a severe 'ice' addiction in his early twenties. He was far from the disadvantaged member of the underclass where amphetamine use was rife. He was the son of a wealthy Cantonese family and worked for a global financial corporation. Jeremy started using "ice" every few days, and his illicit consumption started to coincide with seeing a particular prostitute in a Sydney brothel. He said the prostitute started giving the drugs to him as a sex aid but before long she was charging an extra fee for the drug. Within a few months he was a fully fledged addict and arrived to work withdrawing from the drug's effects. His performance was in freefall. He received a warning about not meeting his targets at work. His Chinese parents were in shock.

Jeremy had used marijuana occasionally in his late teens and tried drugs like ecstasy, but they had never been a problem. But he did suffer separation anxiety as a child and described himself as something of a loner in high school. He had a small group of friends and a tremendous fear of interacting with new people. He arrived under my care after taking a break from his job and was considering a career change. He loved baking and was contemplating an apprenticeship. The celebrity pastry chef Adriano Zumbo was his idol.

While in the clinic, Jeremy rarely left his room except for when it was time to attend the addiction groups. He would occasionally ask the nurses for a tablet of Valium to help calm him before facing the scrutiny of other people. It didn't take a genius to see he suffered a serious case of social anxiety. The amphetamines loosened his inhibitions so he could connect with others to the point where a mild-mannered, spiky-haired Chinese boy trained as an accountant was now out of control using prostitutes and amphetamines.

What was interesting during our sessions was that Jeremy showed few changes in his emotional expression. He was always upbeat even while talking about how his life was spiralling out of control. When the emotional expression, what psychiatrists call 'affect', is out of step with the content of the thoughts, it is often a sign of pathological coping. The behaviour is common in people with drug addiction for as a group they tend to be poor at communicating distress effectively and resort to substances. They also lack skills in tolerating frustration and controlling impulses.

Jeremy had two siblings who also suffered mental illness. I organised a meeting with the parents who were overwhelmed with self-blame, wondering what they had done wrong. There was no other family history of mental illness, but Jeremy described a household of emotional constriction and strict application towards studies and academic success. But this could describe the vast majority of Asian households, very few of which led to children suffering mental illness and addiction. I was aware of the Confucian philosophy of a strict devotion to family, filial ties and the stigma of losing face, but this was not enough to explain Jeremy's case. What was more likely was that Jeremy had limited ties or identification to his Chinese ancestry and suffered some of the identity disturbance more common in children of ethnic descent. American studies of addiction in ethnic groups show people who identify strongly with their cultural heritage were less likely to become addicted to drugs, illustrating community ties acted as protective factors.

People have always used drugs and looked for ways to escape the drudgery of our lives. Like most of my generation, I have tried all the usual substances, but was too cautious to partake in anything regularly. Mine was a generation that lacked the social movements or the great wars that unified populations, instead resorting to mind-altering chemicals backed by a thumping soundtrack to give a fleeting sense of transcendence and communal ritual.

The presence of psychoactive drugs in all societies has been simultaneously met with a need to regulate its use, as psychiatrist Theodore Dalrymple writes in his book *Romancing Opiates*:

> Man's desire to take mind-altering substances is as old as society itself: as are attempts to regulate their consumption. If intoxication in one form or another is inevitable, then so is customary or legal restraint upon that intoxication.

As I write this, Filipino President Rodrigo Duterte has launched a campaign to rid the country's streets of the narcotics trade. This campaign has reached a stage where addicts are being killed as a solution to the drug problem rather than treated. The strategy has echoes of Chairman Mao, who killed drug dealers and addicts as part of his revolutionary program against opium use. The irony is that Mao arguably cured more addicts than anyone in history. Addiction can hardly be a typical disease if such threat of punishment can cure it. Nobody ever cured tuberculosis or pneumonia by threatening to jail the patient.

As a clinician it is difficult to see patients like Jeremy and Lynne and not be affected by their suffering and their desire to stop. I have never viewed addiction purely as a disease but as a mix of voluntary choice with physical and moral consequences, interwoven with a strong physiological basis that could overwhelm the minority of susceptible people. Even drugs like heroin do not cause addiction in most people. Likewise, the majority of people who overcome addictions do so with no formal treatment.

When the pharmaceutical company Bayer invented the drug heroin, having purified it from morphine, and brought it to market in 1898, they did not consider its potential for addiction. They sold it as a cough suppressant, which made sense at the time because two of the most lethal diseases were pneumonia and tuberculosis. None of the people they tested heroin on became addicted. In fact, Bayer marketed heroin as a "cure" for morphine addiction.

Much like advocacy in mental health, medicine has gone too far in attempting to reduce the stigma of addiction by enthusiastically promoting the medical model that drug problems are pure diseases. Canadian neuroscientist Professor Marc Lewis, himself a former heroin addict, illustrates in his book The Biology of Desire that the brains of addicts do change, especially the pathways that control reward and pleasure, but that the brain is always changing anyway.

Lewis argues that addiction is best seen as a result of learning pathways being thwarted and hijacked – more a bad habit than disease. Desire is central to the process and he writes, "addiction can only be beaten by the alignment of desire with personally derived, future oriented goals", something Lewis believes the medical model is poorly equipped to accomplish. Addiction is a confidence trick exploiting the natural characteristic of our brains to form repetitive patterns, be it brushing our teeth or riding a bike. Lewis compared addiction to love affairs and found that "they share many psychological and neurological features. Both addictions and love affairs are ignited by attraction – highly rewarding until they cause more trouble than they're worth."

A good way to think about addiction is that it's a special kind of voluntary activity in people with poor coping behaviours. Harvard psychologist Gene Heyman expands on this idea in his book *Addiction: A Disorder of Choice* where he writes that "voluntary activities vary systematically as a function of their consequences, where the consequences include benefits, costs and values". He cites cases of doctors and airline pilots who are reported to their professional bodies and then monitored closely over several years. Their rates of recovery are higher than the average because they have a great deal to lose in terms of jobs, income and status. Courts that stipulate a strict treatment plan instead of sending drug offenders to jail are also more successful. The stick is the threat of going to jail if they don't stay drug free and co-operate with their treatment, while the carrot is the prospect of being free of charges if able to complete the recommended plan. Such approaches incorporate a sophisticated view of human nature combining a moral aspect with a psychological basis. Contingencies are critical to voluntariness.

No level of punishment or reinforcement can alter a behavior if it were entirely an automatic, biological condition. It's not that people actively choose self-destruction, but how many people choose to be fat? Like being overweight, addiction results from the incremental build-up of multiple decisions over a long period of time, usually in the form of reducing some kind of pain or distress in the short term as opposed to taking on the much harder process of confronting larger problems or inadequacies.

At the lay level, the sales pitch of making people believe that addiction and mental illness is a brain condition has been successful. Patients like Lynne and Jeremy ask if there is a brain scan or test that could isolate the section where any problem might lie. There isn't, of course, but this kind of thinking can limit how much patients take on the responsibility of doing the hard, painful work in confronting their psychological weaknesses.

There is a risk that being enthralled to neuroscience means the more we learn about the brain mechanics of a problem, the more we are likely to call it a disease. Yale Professor Sally Satel writes in an article titled "Addiction and Freedom" that, "...reconciling advances in brain science with their meaning for personal, legal, and civic notions of agency and responsibility will be one of our next major cultural projects".

Reducing Lynne's use of prescription drugs was a drawn out process. She fought every reduction in the dose of either her codeine or Valium and often sent long emails about how distressed she was. Meanwhile the expectations of her as a matriarch remained, running around with the children, cooking elaborate meals on Jewish holidays and maintaining appearances within the tight-knit Orthodox community. She continued to feel emotionally neglected by her husband, just as she did by her mother as a child. Here is one of the emails she sent after a session with me:

> I guess when it rains it pours. I can't stop crying from the pain in my head and emotionally what this brings me to is me debilitated and not being able to live up to any standard never mind an expectation I feel like such a loser like when is this nightmare all going to end? I feel like my life has taken a pathway of difficulty that is beyond my ability to deal with and it scares me that I am going to be like this forever. I know I cant judge myself in this current state but this current state is yet another manifestation of my helplessness or at least that's how I feel right now. Besides for the physical pain I feel physically and emotionally paralysed by everything I dont know how I became like this or how to get out of this rut. Maybe its just the migraine wearing me down bc I was doing well but what if its not. Im sick of my life being like this I dont know how to help myself anymore. Can you help me? Please? I'm so lost.

Her desperation was palpable but she was also beginning to show some insight that her pain might have psychological origins. Her underlying perfectionism and the contradiction of her self-image as highly capable and beautiful was at odds with the current reality, which drove some of her avoidance behaviours. There were days where she lay in bed. Like all addicts, there was a psychic wound that lay below the stupor induced by the substances.

Every reduction of her codeine or benzodiazepine was like pulling teeth. She would fight it. Was there another way? Could we go slower, doctor? Maybe not this week?

She tried everything, but in the end she went along with whatever I suggested. There was no question of her suffering. Her headaches worsened. Her husband described her body shaking, usually while lying in bed. She'd been through every conceivable test over the years and other illnesses like epilepsy had been excluded. Her worst days were after attending synagogue. That was when she had to interact with the Orthodox community. She was understandably wary of being a victim of gossip and innuendo, but she showed strength in facing the crowds and scrutiny.

Lynne felt like an outsider, almost in exile and in fear of being shunned. Her mindset was a symbol of the Jewish historical experience more generally. But her progress was a clear indicator that she had accepted a calculation. In spite of her huge cravings for codeine to minimise the pain she experienced, she could no longer accept the damage her addiction was doing to her children and the potential it had to dissolve her marriage. Divorce would have far greater stigma in her circles than in the broader community. She had cut her losses and made a voluntary choice, but with the guidance of experts.

With Jeremy, it was early days but he was able to remain abstinent. My suggestion regarding his career was that he should wait till he made further improvements and reconsider his current job, of which he had expressed dissatisfaction. He complained about the office politics and how annoying the status and power games were, citing some stories of backstabbing and strategic office romances. But while he was a patient in hospital, he also complained about the frustration he felt about interacting with other patients, especially the trivial and banal conversation. For all the tedium that small talk could be, it was a necessary social dance, and I deduced Jeremy's frustrations had more to do with his problems with interacting socially.

Fearing rejection and humiliation by others, he projected his disaffection upon them. The frustration he felt was his own angst about his capabilities. Many of my patients had a tendency to blame their problems on external aspects of their lives, such as their job, their house or their relationship. While this was the actual reason in some cases, the source for the majority was in their own self image and coping behaviours.

Patients like Lynne and Jeremy are from privileged groups with money and education, but for both of them their psychological skills threatened to destroy their opportunities and social foundations. When I see patients from more disadvantaged backgrounds, their difficulties in climbing the social ladder are rarely to do with money, but to do with psychological habits, namely problems with impulse control, tolerating frustration and maintaining application in pursuing long term goals. There is inevitably a history of instability, neglect or abuse in their childhood. Family life is invariably fragmented. There is also nowhere the level of stigma or shame around drug use or promiscuity that Lynne's or Jeremy's social environment may have. This has its positives, given stigma and shame can lead to greater levels of denial and secrecy, but if there were no negative consequences there were few social disincentives to problematic behaviours.

An influential book about addiction in recent years is by British journalist Johann Hari, the author of *Chasing The Scream*. Hari travels the world interviewing addicts, experts and policy makers. His key point is that drugs aren't the cause of addiction, but the inability to connect with others in meaningful relationships is. He makes reference to a rat experiment in which the rats stop using drugs when they have a social environment to engage with.

This is not exactly a newsflash to anybody working in addiction, but Hari's point about there being a psychic wound limiting relationships is sound. Like Jeremy, in particular, our most urgent need is to connect to others, love, feel loved and be able to engage in purposeful, useful activity. When our coping responses thwart this aim, we are more vulnerable to the escape and elixir of substances.

Hari also writes at length about how the so-called 'war on drugs' has failed. This is more an American than Australian trend. In my experience with patients and the courts, I have never seen a patient go to jail on account of their personal use of drugs. In Australia, much like Britain, we go out of our way to allow people to use drugs for personal use. You only have to look at injecting rooms, needle exchanges and methadone programs. Public psychiatric ward in hospitals are teeming with people admitted after becoming paranoid or threatening after using drugs like amphetamines. Instead of arresting them, the police drive their vans straight to the admissions sections of mental health departments. The problem is usually that if people start becoming serious addicts, they are more likely to start dealing to help pay for their own consumption.

One of the most famous psychological exercises in history is known as the 'marshmallow experiment'. It was conducted at Stanford University in the 1960s. Pre-school children were tempted with marshmallows to eat now or receive larger ones if they could wait more than fifteen minutes. They were then interviewed many years later.

The exercise demonstrated that those who could delay gratification at age eight and not grab the marshmallow in front of them performed better in both relationships and career. I can't think of too many adults who could avoid grabbing the marshmallow in front of them, let alone eight year olds, but the lesson has never been more relevant.

We have never had greater access to cheap, stimulating activities that give us short bursts of pleasure. I have one patient who is addicted to both pornography and gambling. With the advent of the smartphone, he is able to watch porn and bet at the same time. He said it was like playing the poker machines while being entertained by strippers, a scenario that was akin to Nirvana. He once placed a bet on Race 8 in Moonee Valley while in the waiting room of my clinic.

This particular phase of addiction history and the perils of poor impulse control are explored in British philosopher Avner Offer's book, *The Challenge of Affluence*. Some of the personal traits that we might have called good character, like self-control and restraint, have never been more important. The winners of the marshmallow experiment stand to inherit the Earth. Offer also writes that our prosperity speeds the flow of this novelty, causing a social disorientation and diluting the informal norms and commitment devices that emerge more gradually when change is slow. This is a reference to the scaffolding that families, communities and social stigma used to influence.

This disorientation is my observation in treating patients from the microcosm of the consulting room. But the affluence Offer makes reference to applies, in part, to the groups that were previously poor. While they are still poor in relative terms, they are very wealthy by historical standards and can easily access cheap novelties like fatty food and most drugs. But not only do they lack the funds to access more expensive treatments like drug rehabilitation, they are less likely to have developed the psychological skills to withstand the temptations of modern novelties. This is where the broader cultural trends around self fulfilment through the satiation of individual desires are most detrimental to the poor.

Eventually the geographical challenges that Lynne encountered in seeing me took their toll. I stopped treating her when it became too difficult for her to attend appointments and still manage her considerable family and religious obligations. She had made considerable advances in a relatively short period, less than six months, but the challenges she faced were considerable. I think of her regularly, particularly if I visit the area of Sydney where many Orthodox Jews are noticeable in the street, bearded men all dressed in black. I imagine her standing next to her husband in synagogue, perhaps in pain and craving medication. I imagine her toiling away for many guests and visitors and walking long distances during Jewish holidays when it was forbidden for her to drive.

Jeremy was proving a success. When he last consulted me he had left his well-paid job and begun a baking course. I was shocked but impressed by his resolve. Several weeks had passed since he'd completed the inpatient rehabilitation program and he had not once used amphetamines. The prostitute he previously visited contacted him on several occasions, and despite being tempted he was able to resist.

Addiction remains baffling at times and striking the right balance of being caring and firm is a work in progress for me. I found what was most useful was being empathetic and allowing addicts to think of addiction as a disease in the early phase of their treatment. This also helped get people in the door of treatment programs. But once I was able to form a strong therapeutic relationship with the patient and engage important family members in the treatment process, it was then a degree of bad cop and a stronger focus on clear goals with both carrots and sticks was effective. An element of this approach exists across the board in all mental health cases, highlighting that we are complex creatures with a combination of moral and psychological elements. Treating addicts like fragile victims of disease disempowers them and helps no one.

# CONCLUSION

The response I get when introducing myself as a psychiatrist is never neutral. Either people are repulsed and concerned that I am diagnosing them with a mental illness or they are enthralled that they may extract a free consultation. Some expect me to have a beard and Jewish sounding name. Few people have a clear idea of our modern role.

This isn't a surprise given its intellectual edifice is much weaker than other medical disciplines. But its influence is arguably much greater, crossing into welfare, popular culture, disability and the law.

This book is an observation of the cultural rise of mental health through the eyes of my patients. Their extraordinary array of responses to emotional distress illustrate that our minds defy easy categorization. I also wrote the book because I felt there were influences external to my consulting room, from compensation to welfare to social attitudes, that made it more difficult to help my patients.

The patients themselves represents a slice of multicultural Australia in all its diversity and dynamism. The book is not a call to arms or a cry of crisis. Australia is one of the most prosperous, cohesive and peaceful societies in the world. Just as in other issues, in mental health we sit somewhere between the emotional containment of Britain and the flair for psychic expression that characterizes Americans.

But the modern condition is increasingly one of anxiety, particularly around the governance of the soul, of managing the project of individual self-fulfillment. We have shifted from a concern of managing the ego, with its emphasis on regulating desire within the confines of civilization, to a greater focus on self.

Many presentations in the setting of mental health are about excessive individual pre-occupation, a belief that the better one gets in touch with authentic feelings the more likely the path to meaning. As illustrated through my cases, this is influenced by the prevailing culture. My job is often to help steer people to realize the self is realised through our interactions and relationships with others and in the exercise of useful, purposeful activity.

Mental health promotion influences our conceptions of human nature. Our disruptive times are in part related to shifting views and battles about what constitutes our nature as traditional structures of authority disintegrate.

Few clinical specialists apply a mechanistic or bureaucratic version of practice, but mental health promotion has sold a view of people whose emotional distress is caused either by their biology or the outside world. This is worsened by the loosening of the definition of terms like trauma which is changing our relationship to adversity and our sensitivity to harm.

While such promotion helps reduce stigma, the risk is the field is contributing to the current political challenges of either resentment based movements or passive disengagement of large swathes of the population. The decline of religion and the rise of positive psychology also contribute to an overly optimistic view of our natures, leading to people being less able to cope with difficult, dark emotions.

The aim of the psychological sciences was to help people achieve greater self-knowledge into their own coping behaviours so as to better handle the challenges of living in society. This helps people manage relationships leading to better families, societies and workplaces. Psychology cannot entirely replace the ethics and values that systems like religion gave us. We remain moral beings. We are also fundamentally resilient and constructing vulnerability on a large scale limits recovery and empowerment.

# ACKNOWLEDGEMENTS

The stories are based on my experience and recollections of patients. Names and details have been changed. All are inspiring in their utmost courage in the face of great suffering. Thanks also to the staff and colleagues who help me care for them and offer their experience and wisdom.

An obvious but important thank you goes to the publisher Connor Court and its powerhouse in Anthony Cappello. The concept of this book was not entirely developed and the writing of the original two cases pitched to several publishers was, in hindsight, lacking in direction. Anthony effectively took a gamble and allowed me to find my voice and style, with the help of excellent, generous editor Glenda Downing.

I must make special mention to my supporters in the media and cultural worlds. They know who they are and without them I would have struggled to retain a voice and involvement in the public sphere. Several of them read the manuscript and offered advice, feedback and testimonials. I am very grateful in their faith in my work.

My final thank you are to my wonderful family: my parents and relatives have provided support and nourishment in innumerable ways. My beautiful, brilliant wife, Alina Hughes, who has been the ground beneath my feet for sixteen years and our two divine children – Katarina and Saskia – who enrich our lives every day.

# REFERENCES

## 1

Ahmed, Tanveer, 2005, "The Muslim 'Marginal Man'", *Policy*, Vol. 21, No. 1, Autumn 2005

Roy, Olivier 2004, *Globalised Islam : the search for a new Ummah*, Hurst, London

Hermansen, Marcia , "How to Put the Genie back in the Bottle: Identity Islam and Muslim Youth Cultures in the United States", in Omid Safi (ed.) *Progressive Muslims: On Pluralism, Gender, and Justice* (Oxford: Oneworld Publications, 2003)

Mishra, Pankaj 2006, *Temptations of the West : how to be modern in India, Pakistan and beyond*, Picador, London

Patai, Raphael 2002, *The Arab mind, Rev. ed*, Hatherleigh Press, New York, N.Y.

## 2

*TIME Magazine*, February 1965, "Psychiatry: Homosexuals Can Be Cured"

## 3

This is an adapted article from one I wrote for the *Griffith Review 45* titled Trauma, Work and Adversity in their The Way We Work edition.

Watters, Ethan 2010, *Crazy like us : the globalisation of the American psyche*, Scribe, Carlton North, Vic

Dean, Eric T 1997, *Shook over hell : post-traumatic stress, Vietnam, and the Civil War*, Harvard University Press, Cambridge, Mass

Young, Allan 1995, The harmony of illusions : inventing post-traumatic stress disorder, Princeton University Press, Princeton, N.J

Wessely, S. (2005) 'Risk, psychiatry and the military', *The British Journal of Psychiatry*, 186, 459-466.

4

Taylor, Charles & Taylor, Charles. Malaise of modernity 1992, *The ethics of authenticity*, Harvard University Press, Cambridge, Mass

Elliott, Carl 2003, *Better than well : American medicine meets the American dream*, W.W. Norton, New York

Cederström, Carl & Spicer, André, (author.) 2015, *The Wellness Syndrome*, *Cambridge*, UK Malden, MA Polity

Biss, Eula 2015, *On immunity : an inoculation*, Melbourne, Victoria, The Text Publishing Company

5

Brooks, David 2015, *The road to character*, New York Random House

Martin, Mike W & Oxford University Press 2006, *From morality to mental health : virtue and vice in a therapeutic culture*, Oxford University Press, Oxford

Goldhill, Olivia, "An Oxford neuroethicist on how drugs can make us more moral". *Quartz magazine*. August 20, 2016.

Kramer, Peter D 1993, *Listening to Prozac*, Viking, New York, N.Y., U.S.A

Karen Blixen as quoted to Hanna Arendt in *The Human Condition* (1958).

6

I have partially adapted this chapter from my *Spectator Australia* column titled "White Noise", January 23, 2016.

Douthat, Ross Gregory & Salam, Reihan 2008, *Grand new party : how republicans can win the working class and save the American dream*, Doubleday, New York

O'Hagan, Andrew, "The annual Orwell Memorial Lecture at Birkbeck College", November 13, 2008, YouTube

Kimmell, Michael, 2014, *Angry White Men: American Masculinity at the End of an*

*Era,* Nation Books, New York

Davies, Will, 2016, "Thoughts on the Sociology of Brexit. Political Economy Research Centre", http://www.perc.org.uk/project_posts/thoughts-on-the-sociology-of-brexit/

7

Uribe Guajardo, Maria Gabriela & Slewa-Younan, Shameran & Smith, Mitchell & Eagar, Sandy & Stone, Glenn 2016-01-20, 'Psychological distress is influenced by length of stay in resettled Iraqi refugees in Australia.(Report)' *International Journal of Mental Health Systems,* vol. 10, no. 4

Watters, Ethan 2011, *Crazy like us,* Robinson, London

Horwitz, Allan V & Wakefield, Jerome C 2007, *The loss of sadness : how psychiatry transformed normal sorrow into depressive disorder,* Oxford University Press, Oxford; New York

My *Spectator Australia* column "I'm An Asylum Seeker, Get Me Out of Here" February 13, 2016.

One of the patients profiled posted part of his email sent to me on a site called Drugs.com. He did so under a pseudonym.

8

Phone interview conducted with Dr John Collier, August 30, 2016

Phone interview conducted with Jenny Alum, September 29, 2016

Baumeister, Roy & Campbell, Jennifer D & Krueger, Joachim I & Vohs, Kathleen D, "Exploding the Self Esteem Myth", ScientificAmerican.com, December 20, 2004, https://www.uvm.edu/~wgibson/PDF/Self-Esteem%20Myth.pdf

Turkle, Sherry 2011, *Alone together : why we expect more from technology and less from each other,* Basic, New York

9

The chapter is adapted from a short story I wrote first published in a site I co-founded bddiaspora.com

Coontz, Stephanie 2005, *Marriage, a history : from obedience to intimacy or how love conquered marriage,* New York Viking

Sandhu, Sukhdev, "Come Hungry, leave edgy". *London Review of Books,* October 2003

10

Dalrymple, Theodore 2008, *Romancing opiates : pharmacological lies and the addiction bureaucracy,* Encounter, New York

Lewis, Marc 2015, *The biology of desire : why addiction is not a disease,* Brunswick, Victoria Scribe Publications

Heyman, Gene M 2009, *Addiction : a disorder of choice,* Harvard University Press, Cambridge, Mass

Satel, Sally, "Addiction and Freedom", *New Republic,* March 2010

Hari, Johann 2015, *Chasing the scream : the first and last days of the war on drugs,* London Bloomsbury Circus

Offer, Avner 2006, *The challenge of affluence : self-control and well-being in the United States and Britain since 1950,* Oxford University Press, Oxford